Contents

Supplements for Endurance Athletes

Jose Antonio, PhD, CSCS, FACSM
Jeffrey R. Stout, PhD, CSCS*D, FACSM

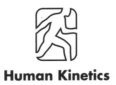

Human Kinetics

Library of Congress Cataloging-in-Publication Data

Antonio, Jose, PhD.
    Supplements for endurance athletes / by Jose Antonio, Jeffrey R. Stout.
        p. cm.
    Includes bibliographical references.
    ISBN 0-7360-3773-X
    1. Dietary supplements. 2. Endurance sports. 3.
Athletes--Nutrition. I. Stout, Jeffrey R. II. Title.
    RM258.5 .A57 2002

                                        2002002999

ISBN: 0-7360-3773-X

Copyright © 2002 by Human Kinetics Publishers, Inc.

Acquisitions Editor: Michael S. Barhke, PhD; **Developmental Editor:** D.K. Bihler; **Assistant Editor:** Lee Alexander; **Copyeditor:** Scott J. Weckerly; **Proofreader:** Sue Fetters; **Permission Manager:** Dalene Reeder; **Graphic Designer:** Nancy Rasmus; **Graphic Artist:** Dawn Sills; **Photo Manager:** Leslie A. Woodrum; **Cover Designer:** Keith Blomberg; **Photographer (cover):** David Madison Sports Images Inc.; **Art Manager:** Carl D. Johnson; **Illustrator:** Tom Roberts; **Printer:** United Graphics

Printed in the United States of America   10 9 8 7 6 5 4 3 2 1

Human Kinetics
Web site: www.humankinetics.com

United States: Human Kinetics
P.O. Box 5076
Champaign, IL 61825-5076
800-747-4457
e-mail: humank@hkusa.com

Australia: Human Kinetics
57A Price Avenue
Lower Mitcham, South Australia 5062
08 8277 1555
e-mail: liahka@senet.com.au

Canada: Human Kinetics
475 Devonshire Road Unit 100
Windsor, ON N8Y 2L5
800-465-7301 (in Canada only)
e-mail: orders@hkcanada.com

New Zealand: Human Kinetics
P.O. Box 105-231, Auckland Central
09-523-3462
e-mail: hkp@ihug.co.nz

Europe: Human Kinetics
107 Bradford Road
Stanningley
Leeds LS28 6AT, United Kingdom
+44 (0) 113 255 5665
e-mail: hk@hkeurope.com

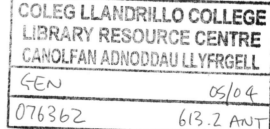

Preface

Do you have visions of finishing the New York City marathon? (Remember that's 26.2 miles!) Or, if you have finished a marathon before, wouldn't it be great if you could finish it just a little bit faster? If so, then you need to read this book.

Or how about this scenario: You're a Division I, collegiate middle-distance runner and you're starting to feel tired, lethargic, and listless. It's one of those days when you step on the track, mentally preparing yourself for doing repeat 400s with 200-meter rest intervals, and it's painfully apparent that you just don't have the energy. Perhaps you're not getting enough calories. Or maybe you're skimping on the protein. Would something like glutamine, a conditionally essential amino acid, help you? If you're not sure, then this book is definitely for you.

What exactly is this book about, and who is it for? This is the second book in a two-part series on dietary supplements for athletes. Although the majority of supplements are targeted toward strength-power athletes, there is a growing body of evidence that shows that endurance athletes can be helped with specific dietary supplements as well.

Certainly, the importance of carbohydrates during prolonged endurance exercise is clear and well-established. Consuming high-glycemic carbohydrates during continuous exercise lasting two hours or more will probably improve your performance. But we believe that there's more to an endurance athlete's nutrition program than carbohydrates. Though many supplements have no known ergogenic effects for endurance, there are many others that may play a useful role in the dietary repertoire of the endurance athlete.

We admit that more research needs to be done in this area. However, athletes and those who give advice to athletes (nutritionists, exercise physiologists, coaches, and so on) do not necessarily have the time to wait for scientists to come to a consensus on "what works and what doesn't." Instead, there is a mixture of science, trial and error, and just plain intuition

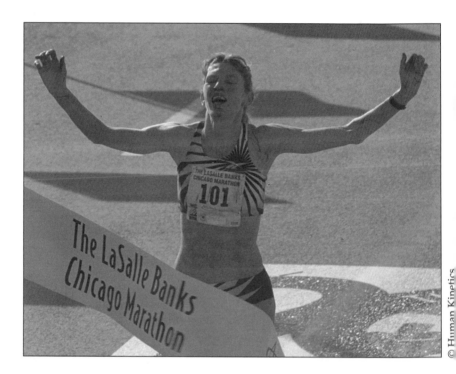

© Human Kinetics

that goes into formulating an eating and supplementation plan for athletes. With limited data and time (the career of many professional athletes rarely spans more than a decade), it is critical that we provide the best information to our knowledge on supplements that may improve endurance performance. To hide behind the notion of "more research is needed" and therefore not offer advice would be nothing less than intellectual laziness.

Our book offers practical information in an easy-to-follow format. Each supplement, presented in alphabetical order by chapter, is explained in five separate subheadings. Also, for those of you who are neophytes to science, we have a glossary of terms that will help you understand our scientific jargon.

- **What Is It?**

  In this section, each supplement is defined in chemical terms.

- **How Does It Work?**

  In this section, we present the theoretical basis for how this supplement may help an endurance athlete.

- **The Evidence: Pro or Con?**

  In this section, we present the latest scientific studies that support or refute the efficacy of a particular supplement.

- **Guidelines for Use**

  In this section, we provide practical advice regarding the potential use of a supplement.

- **Precautions**

  In this section, we briefly mention the possible side effects that a supplement may have.

In addition, we have an easy-to-follow glossary of common terms used in sports nutrition and supplementation as it applies to endurance athletes.

You can skip those sections you find uninteresting and go straight to the bottom line (i.e., Guidelines for Use). We hope, however, that you will find all of the information intriguing and useful. You can either choose to accept our recommendations or not. Though we are trained as research scientists, we also value the "trial and error" information garnered by athletes. While the scientific purist may cringe at the thought of using such anecdotal information, it is often the case that athletes use supplements or combinations of supplements long before science can confirm or deny their benefits.

For instance, we were told as youngsters that eating candy (i.e., sugar, mainly sucrose) would give us "quick energy" for an athletic event. Interestingly, this age-old advice has been confirmed in many studies showing that, indeed, carbohydrate consumption prior and during an endurance-type event will yield performance benefits. Let's say that 50 years ago, a runner had told you that consuming a sugar-containing beverage during a marathon had actually helped him run faster. The science was nonexistent back then. Should we, as scientists, tell him that this was a waste of time? Or should we pay heed to what athletes are actually doing?

It would be foolhardy to ignore the actual dietary practices of athletes. Besides, they're the ones who pay the price for choosing to (or not to) use a particular supplement. It is all too easy for scientists to state that dietary supplements are generally a waste of time and money.

Our book takes findings from the laboratory and attempts to find practical applications for them (if they exist). It is obvious that certain supplements are indeed a waste of time and money, but on the other hand, there are plenty of supplements that endurance athletes may find useful. To ignore this possibility would be parochial and narrow-minded. The purpose of this book is to give athletes the information that is known *right now* so that they can make informed decisions. However, if you choose to use our book—either from cover-to-cover or as an occasional reference—we wish you the best of fortune in your athletic career.

β-Hydroxy-β-Methylbutyrate

What Is It?

β-Hydroxy-β-Methylbutyrate (HMB) is a breakdown product (metabolite) of the amino acid leucine (Nissen et al. 1996). Leucine is found in all dietary protein and is an essential building block of protein in all tissues. Among the amino acids, leucine holds a special place. In addition to being an essential amino acid (one that must be supplied from the diet), it's also one of three amino acids termed *branched-chain amino acids*. Leucine's truly unique characteristic, however, is its role in regulating protein synthesis and protein breakdown.

How Does It Work?

The first clue to understanding the effect of HMB on protein metabolism was research conducted on the first metabolite of leucine, ketoisocaproate (KIC). Researchers found that KIC could duplicate most, if not all, of the effects of leucine in tissues. Early research (Chua, Siehl, and Morgan 1979; Mortimore et al. 1987) found that both leucine and KIC decreased proteolysis (protein breakdown) and increased protein synthesis in isolated tissues. Additional studies found nitrogen sparing (Cerosimo et al. 1983; Mortimore et al. 1987) and reductions in muscle glucose utilization (Buckspan et al. 1986) with KIC in humans subjected to stressful situations. The leucine dose in these studies was about 120 g/day (Cerosimo et al. 1983) and about half that for KIC (Buckspan et al. 1986; Mitch, Walser, and Spair 1981). As a side note, most of these studies were conducted under extreme conditions, such as starvation, trauma, or severe burns.

1

Despite all of the aforementioned research, the data with KIC suggested that the leucine effect was not due to leucine but instead due to a down-stream product. The same question remained: Was the effect due to KIC or some further breakdown product in the pathway, of which there are about eight additional biochemicals? In the early 1980s, scientists proposed an alternative metabolic pathway of leucine metabolism, which indicated that KIC was metabolized by an enzyme distinct to HMB.

Scientists at Iowa State University were the first to test the hypothesis that this HMB metabolite may mediate the effects of leucine and KIC on protein metabolism. Their postulation led them to a series of animal experiments and later to human experiments spanning the last 10 years. These extensive studies indicate that HMB is the bioactive component of leucine metabolism and that it helps regulate protein metabolism (Nissen et al. 1996).

Research in animals and humans suggests that HMB plays a role in protein metabolism as well, especially in stressful situations such as high-intensity running (Knitter et al. 2000). Although no one is certain of the mechanism(s) behind HMB, scientists have been working on two hypotheses (Nissen et al. 1996):

Hypothesis 1. HMB may be an essential component of the cell membrane. Scientists propose that under stressful situations, the body may not make enough HMB to satisfy the increased needs of tissues. It could also be that stress may alter either the enzymes or the concentration of certain biochemicals that decrease normal HMB production. Either scenario would require dietary supplementation of HMB for the skeletal muscle system to maximally function.

Hypothesis 2. HMB may regulate enzymes responsible for muscle tissue breakdown. This theory is supported by the evidence found in several studies in which biochemical indicators of muscle damage were decreased (see the following section for explanation).

The Evidence: Pro or Con?

In most scenarios, high-intensity, long-duration runs can lead to muscle soreness caused by structural damage to skeletal muscle; damage to the muscle can then lead to a reduced physical performance (Knitter et al. 2000). Therefore, if HMB supplementation can decrease protein breakdown usually seen with high-intensity, long-duration running, then the athlete could recover more quickly and HMB would prove to be an effective aid.

Dr. Nissen and colleagues conducted the first human-performance study in 1996 at Iowa State University. In this study, male subjects participated in an exercise-training program and were assigned to either a control group, a group that consumed 1.5 g HMB per day, or a group that consumed 3 g HMB per day. After a one-week adaptation period, the three-week supplementation and exercise protocol started (a total-body, weight-training program). After only one week of training/supplementation, muscle protein breakdown in the group fed 3 g HMB decreased 44% (compared with the placebo group) as measured by 3-methylhistidine (3-MH) loss in urine. (A muscle-specific amino acid, 3-MH is produced and lost in urine only when muscle protein is broken down.)

Muscle protein breakdown continued to be lower in the HMB group for the entire three-week study. A second indicator of muscle damage and muscle breakdown is the muscle-specific enzyme creatine phosphokinase (CPK). This enzyme was also markedly decreased with HMB supplementation.

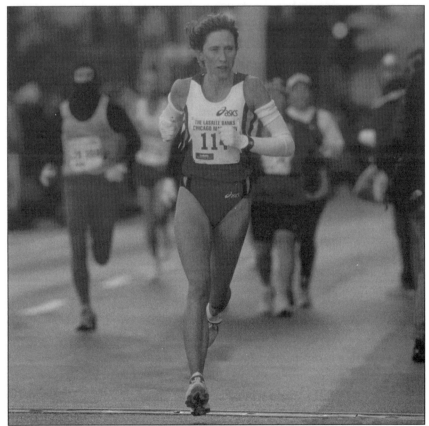

© Human Kinetics

In a more recent study (Knitter et al. 2000) using highly trained male and female runners, scientists determined whether HMB could reduce muscle damage after a long-distance run. The endurance athletes were paired into two groups based on their two-mile run time. In a random, double-blind design, one group received 3 g HMB per day while the other group received a placebo. After six weeks of supplementation and training, both groups participated in a 20 K run. Four days after exercise, the group taking 3 g HMB per day experienced 25% less muscle damage as measured by CPK activity levels (see figure 1.1). The authors concluded that HMB supplementation helped to prevent exercise-induced muscle damage from high-intensity, long-duration running.

In another endurance study, Vukovich and Adams (1997) studied the effects of HMB on highly trained cyclists. Eight cyclists randomly supplemented daily for two weeks with either a placebo, 3 g leucine, or 3 g HMB. Prior to and immediately following supplementation period, the subjects underwent a $\dot{V}O_2$max test, which tests cardiovascular fitness (endurance). (The higher the $\dot{V}O_2$max value, the more likely your performance will be better.) The HMB supplementation period resulted in a significant increase in $\dot{V}O_2$max when compared with the placebo and leucine supplementation (see figure 1.2). Researchers therefore concluded that HMB supplementation may have a positive effect on endurance performance.

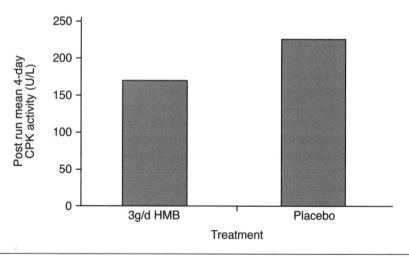

Figure 1.1 Effect of HMB supplementation on muscle damage after a long run. Data from Knitter et al. 2000.

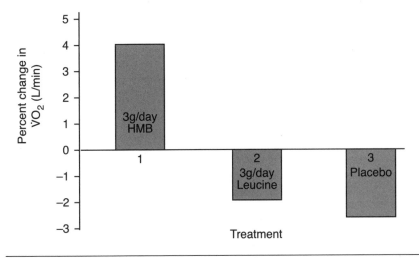

Figure 1.2 Effect of HMB supplementation on $\dot{V}O_2$max. Data from Vukovich and Adams 1997.

Guidelines for Use

As you can see, HMB is an interesting dietary supplement that may benefit the endurance athlete. Exactly how effective this supplement is remains to be seen, but what we know so far is intriguing. An effective dose appears to be 3 g/day (Gallagher et al. 2000a, 2000b; Nissen et al. 1996; Vukovich and Adams 1997).

Precautions

As we mentioned, the recommended dose is 3 g/day, and no adverse effects are expected at 3 g/day. In addition, studies ranging from one to eight weeks have demonstrated that even up to 6 g/day is safe and well tolerated (Gallagher et al. 2000a, 2000b; Nissen et al. 2000).

Branched-Chain Amino Acids

What Are They?

The branched-chain amino acids (BCAA) are composed of leucine, valine, and isoleucine. BCAA are essential amino acids that your body cannot synthesize; thus, you need to acquire them from your diet. BCAA are found in high concentrations in whey protein. In addition, you'll find them in meats, fish, milk, eggs, and other quality protein sources.

How Do They Work?

One of the underlying reasons for supplementing with BCAA is the fact that they are catabolized during endurance-type exercise (especially leucine) (Hargreaves and Snow 2001). For instance, in a carbohydrate-depleted state, such as during four hours of continuous exercise, alanine is made in skeletal muscles from pyruvate and amino acids (especially the BCAA). Alanine leaves the skeletal muscle cells, enters the circulation, and goes to the liver where it is converted to glucose. Glucose then leaves the liver and is delivered to muscle for use as fuel. The BCAA can be used by skeletal muscle during exercise, as well.

Besides providing additional energy, BCAA supplementation during a long-endurance event competes with tryptophan (an amino acid precursor to serotonin) for entry into the central nervous system (the brain). How does this reaction affect fatigue? Scientists have theorized that tryptophan elevates levels of the brain neurotransmitter serotonin, or 5-hydroxytryptamine (5-HTP). If BCAA predominates the brain over tryptophan, they would offset fatigue.

In other words, BCAA may help athletes avoid what is called central fatigue (mental fatigue) during and after prolonged exercise. For instance, athletes often complain of that drowsy, lethargic feeling after a two-hour run or bike ride. That fatigue may be due to high levels of 5-HTP. Athletes can offset the increase in 5-HTP by consuming BCAA because BCAA and tryptophan compete for entry into the brain. When you get tryptophan into the brain, it enhances serotonin synthesis and, therefore, feelings of fatigue. If you can decrease the amount of tryptophan by ingesting BCAA, then the end result is less fatigue after a long workout.

The Evidence: Pro or Con?

Studies done on BCAA have arrived at different conclusions—some positive for endurance athletes, some not, and some intriguing nevertheless. In one study, Blomstrand et al. (1995) had five male endurance-trained

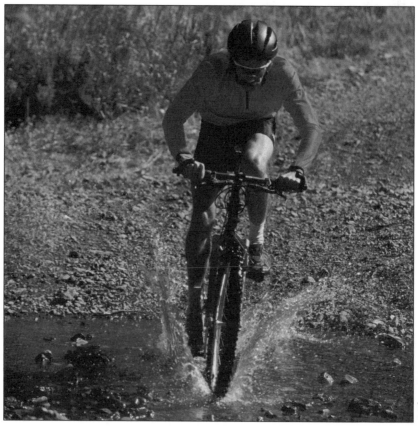

© PhotoDisc

subjects cycle at 75% $\dot{V}O_2$max until exhaustion. During exercise, the subjects were randomly given one of the following: a flavored water solution (placebo), a 6% carbohydrate solution with 7 g/L BCAA, or a 6% carbohydrate solution without BCAA.

Performance decreased in four out of the five subjects during the flavored water trial when compared with the two carbohydrate periods. However, no differences in performance were seen between the two carbohydrate groups. In this case, adding BCAA to carbohydrate had no further effect on performance. In agreement with these findings, other scientists have also failed to show an ergogenic effect of BCAA consumption (Blomstrand et al. 1997; Struder et al. 1998; Van Hall et al. 1995).

Not all studies are negative with regards to BCAA use, however. In one study, the consumption of BCAA during a marathon (26.2 miles) improved performance for the slower runners (3.05 hours and longer) whereas it had no effect on the faster runners (under 3.05 hours) (Blomstrand et al. 1991). In a study from Rutgers University, six men and seven women ingested either a placebo or 5 ml/kg body weight (about 2.3 ml/lb) of a BCAA drink every 30 minutes during cycle exercise (40% $\dot{V}O_2$ peak to exhaustion) in the heat (34 °C) (Mittleman et al. 1998). The BCAA-consuming group lasted 11.7% longer on the bike (see figure 2.1). During the BCAA trial, the women on average consumed a total of 9.4 g BCAA while the men consumed 15.8 g (see figure 2.2). The majority of the amino acid consumed was leucine.

Interestingly, BCAA may help recovery via their effect on reducing muscle damage as a result of exercise. In a study from the University of Tasmania (Coombes and McNaughton 2000), 16 male subjects consumed 12 g BCAA daily for 14 days in addition to their normal diet (a control

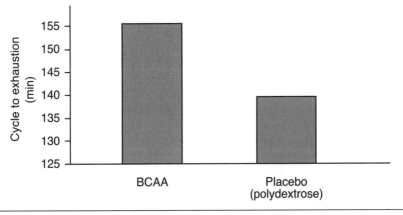

Figure 2.1 Effect of BCAA on time to exhaustion. Data from Mittleman et al. 1998.

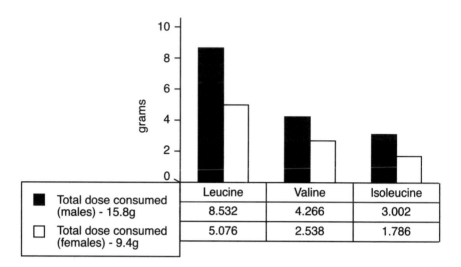

	Leucine	Valine	Isoleucine
■ Total dose consumed (males) - 15.8g	8.532	4.266	3.002
☐ Total dose consumed (females) - 9.4g	5.076	2.538	1.786

Figure 2.2 BCAA formula: Ergogenic effects during moderate exercise in the heat. Data from Mittleman et al. 1998.

group consumed a normal diet only). On the seventh day, subjects took part in an exercise test (cycle at 70% of $\dot{V}O_2$max for 120 minutes). Blood samples were taken postexercise at 1 hour, 2 hours, 3 hours, 4 hours, 1 day, 3 days, 5 days, and 7 days. Diets were analyzed on day 14. They found that all subjects consumed the recommended daily BCAA intake in their normal diets (0.64 g/kg body weight daily, about 0.29 g/lb). Even without supplementation, the placebo group consumed enough BCAA to meet basic requirements.

But what is intriguing about this study is that the BCAA-supplemented group had lower blood levels of lactate dehydrogenase (LDH) from two hours to five days postexercise and lower levels of creatine kinase (CK) from four hours to five days postexercise. (LDH and CK are enzymes that "leak" from damaged muscle cells. Elevated levels of these enzymes indicate injury to muscle fibers.) This study indicates that supplementing with BCAA may reduce muscle damage, which results from endurance exercise.

BCAA may further reduce the protein breakdown associated with resistance-type endurance exercises. In one study, five men performed single-leg knee extensions for 60 minutes at 71% maximal work capacity with or without BCAA supplementation (77 mg/kg body weight; about 5.77 g BCAA for 165-lb person) (MacLean, Graham, and Saltin 1994). Intramuscular BCAA concentrations were higher for the BCAA trial and remained higher throughout the exercise bout. Additionally, the net release of essential amino acids from skeletal muscle was higher in the control group than in the BCAA group, which would indicate that BCAA supplementation may decrease exercise-induced, muscle protein breakdown. Theoretically, then, BCAA consumption may help you recover more quickly than otherwise and help you get back to a normal training routine after a tough bout of exercise.

BCAA supplementation clearly does not harm performance. Unfortunately, it is apparent that the data regarding BCAA are equivocal. In some cases, it has no effects; for others, it helps. Individual differences in biochemistry may determine whether this supplement is effective for you and your particular sport.

Guidelines for Use

If BCAA are to have any effect at all for endurance athletes, they must be taken in doses that are between 9 and 15 g (total dose consumed during exercise of approximately two hours). Alternatively, supplementing with 12 g/day for two weeks may offset some of the muscle damage that results from training.

BCAA have an unpleasant taste when mixed with a drink, so many will avoid their use during an endurance event. However, if you can toughen your palate, regular supplementation may be a way to improve recovery because BCAA help damaged skeletal muscle tissue heal faster. If you can improve recovery and recovery time, then theoretically, you should be able to train harder, more frequently, and ultimately become a better and faster endurance athlete.

A range of 6 to 15 g BCAA taken either before exercise or on a daily basis may improve recovery by lessening muscle protein breakdown and injury postexercise. As an alternative, regular consumption of whey protein, which is high in BCAA, may be a more palatable method to get these important amino acids.

Precautions

There are no toxic side effects associated with BCAA supplementation or consumption. There are, however, anecdotal reports of individuals experiencing gastrointestinal distress (stomach pain, diarrhea) after consuming BCAA.

Caffeine and Ephedrine

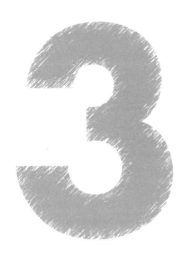

What Are They?

Caffeine is common in our diet and is the most consumed drug in the world. It is unlikely that caffeine's use will decline any time soon—it is inexpensive, medically safe, socially acceptable, and legal (Sinclair and Geinger 2000). Ephedrine is naturally found in the plant genus ephedra or mahuang (Clarkson and Thompson 1997) and is the active ingredient in some over-the-counter oral bronchodilators for the treatment of asthma.

How Do They Work?

Caffeine and ephedrine are believed to affect stimulatory receptors in the central nervous system (CNS), as well as metabolic receptors in peripheral tissues, including skeletal muscles (Bell et al. 1999; Bell et al. 2000). Another hypothesis concerning caffeine and ephedrine as an ergogenic aid is that they enhance fat utilization during exercise, therefore sparing muscle glycogen stores (Chesley et al. 1998; Laurent et al. 2000; Van Soeren and Graham 1998). In addition, caffeine and ephedrine may have the ability to influence psychological states and alter pain perception (Laurent et al. 2000).

The Evidence: Pro or Con?

Although caffeine is usually combined with ephedrine as a potent fat-loss agent, there is an abundance of studies that have examined the role of caffeine (by itself) as a lipolytic agent. In our analysis of the currrent literature, we will first cover studies done on caffeine as a single supplement, then we will follow with a discussion on the combination of caffeine plus ephedrine.

Caffeine Only

One of the first studies to investigate caffeine's effect on exercise metabolism and performance was published by Dr. Costill and colleagues (Costill, Dalsky, and Fink 1978). Subjects consumed decaffeinated coffee or decaffeinated coffee enhanced with 330 mg pure caffeine 60 minutes prior to exercise. Time to exhaustion was over 19% greater in the caffeine trial compared with the decaffeinated trial. The scientists concluded that this increase in performance was likely due to the increase in fat oxidation (using fat for energy). In this study, muscle glycogen (stored form of carbohydrates) was not measured, so they were unable to determine whether caffeine spared muscle glycogen. However, the performance data suggest that the elevation in fat oxidation provided the energy needed for the 19% increase in time to reach exhaustion.

It wasn't until 1987, almost 10 years later, that someone actually investigated the effects of caffeine ingestion on muscle glycogen utilization in humans (Erickson et al. 1987). Caffeine supplementation prior to exercise was found to reduce muscle glycogen utilization by 30%. Subsequent research by Dr. Spriet and coworkers (1992) confirmed Erickson's finding. Dr. Spriet and colleagues reported a 55% decrease in muscle glycogenolysis (use of carbohydrates for energy) in just the first 15 minutes of exercise during the caffeine trial. The decrease in glycogenolysis during the early part of the exercise allowed for more glycogen to be available during the later stages, which resulted in a greater time to exhaustion.

In the first three studies discussed so far, each one has used a different dosage of caffeine: 330 mg (Costill, Dalsky, and Fink 1978), 5 mg/kg (2.3 mg/lb) body weight (Erickson et al. 1987), and 9 mg/kg (4.1 mg/lb) body weight (Spriet et al. 1992). Most of the studies have administered caffeine at a dose of 5 mg/kg of body weight, but the range can be as much as 3.0 to 13 mg/kg (5.9 mg/lb).

To help resolve the question of dosage, two dosing studies have been done to determine which dosage provides the greatest benefit. In the first study, Drs. Graham and Spriet (1995) provided athletes with caffeine at 3, 6, and 9 mg/kg body weight (1.4, 2.7, and 4.1 mg/lb) to determine the effect on exercise metabolism and performance. They reported that the 3 and 6 mg/kg doses both enhanced performance, but the 9 mg/kg dose did not. The 6 and 9 mg/kg doses resulted in elevations in catecholamines (i.e., epinephrine and norepinephrine), and the 9 mg/kg dose resulted in increases in fat catabolism (breakdown). Catecholamines increase metabolism by elevating cardiac output and increasing the rate of glycogen and fat breakdown for energy.

In the second study, Dr. Pasman and coworkers (1995) compared endurance performance with dosages of caffeine at 5, 9, and 13 mg/kg (2.3, 4.1, 5.9 mg/lb) body weight. All three dosages resulted in a significant improvement in endurance performance compared with the placebo trial, but there was no difference among the three dosages of caffeine.

In addition to the dose of caffeine, there are other items that athletes need to be aware of before utilizing caffeine or caffeine-containing products as an ergogenic aid. Habitual caffeine users may respond differently than naïve users (Dodd et al. 1991; Fisher et al. 1986; Tarnopolsky et al. 1989; Van Soeren and Graham 1998). Research indicates that in habitual users, caffeine may increase fat breakdown, but this does not necessarily result in an increase in fat use for energy or an increase in catecholamines or performance. In one study, a four-day withdrawal period resulted in a return of caffeine's effect once caffeine was reintroduced (Fisher et al. 1986). In a more recent study, though, habitual users experienced a significant increase in performance with caffeine supplementation before and after two and four days of withdrawal (Van Soeren and Graham 1998), meaning that its effects worked regardless of the length of withdrawal.

Another factor that should be of interest is the form in which caffeine is consumed. Most research studies use pure caffeine. It is easier to dose, and the purity is known. The general public, however, consumes the majority of caffeine in the form of coffee, not pure caffeine.

To test whether this factor was significant, Graham and colleagues (1998) conducted a study to determine whether coffee produced the same effect as pure caffeine. In a well-designed study, subjects consumed decaffeinated coffee, decaffeinated coffee plus pure caffeine, regular coffee, placebo capsules, or caffeine capsules. The amount of caffeine was the same in all the caffeine trials.

The caffeine capsules resulted in an increase in plasma epinephrine concentration that was greater than all other trials while exercise resulted in an increase in epinephrine in every trial, with no difference between the caffeine conditions. The most interesting aspect of the study is that only the caffeine capsule trial resulted in a significant improvement in performance. Time to exhaustion for the caffeine capsules was 31% greater (9.9 minutes longer) than the placebo capsule trial and 23% greater (7.6 minutes longer) than the decaffeinated trial. The ingestion of caffeinated coffee did not result in an enhancement of performance. The authors concluded that the bioavailability of caffeine is not altered in the form of regular coffee, but that there may be some unknown compounds in coffee that antagonize the effects of caffeine.

Caffeine Plus Ephedrine

It appears that pure caffeine enhances performance, and caffeine-containing products (i.e., coffee, tea) are as yet an undetermined ergogenic aid. To determine whether a combination of caffeine and ephedrine affects athletes, Dr. Bell and colleagues (2000) conducted a study using 12 healthy, untrained male subjects performing high-intensity aerobic exercise. Seven of the subjects consumed caffeine on a regular basis while five were noncaffeine consumers. The subjects ingested either a placebo or a mixture of caffeine and ephedrine in fixed dosages 1.5 to 2.0 hours before exercising. After ingestion, they performed cycle ergometer trials to exhaustion at 85% oxygen consumption ($\dot{V}O_2$).

Oxygen consumption ($\dot{V}O_2$), carbon dioxide production ($\dot{V}CO_2$), and ventilation (V_E) were analyzed every minute by a metabolic cart, which are measurements exercise scientists commonly use to assess cardiovascular fitness and energy expenditure. For example, if $\dot{V}O_2$max goes up, cardiovascular fitness has improved. Heart rate (HR) was also closely monitored throughout every exercise session. The subjects' rate of perceived exertion (RPE) was also measured every five minutes, where they described how hard they thought they were working (i.e., psychological test).

Surprisingly, the combination of caffeine and ephedrine significantly increased the time to exhaustion ride in the caffeine users only; that is, noncaffeine users did not experience a similar effect (see figure 3.1). In

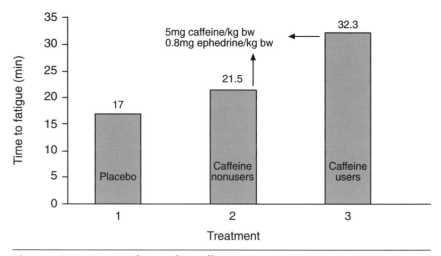

Figure 3.1 Times to fatigue for caffeine users versus nonusers. Data adapted from Bell et al. 2000.

other words, those who consumed caffeine on a regular basis were able to perform the exhaustion ride longer whereas noncaffeine users, despite the caffeine-ephedrine supplement, did not ride as long. $\dot{V}O_2$, $\dot{V}CO_2$, and V_E measurements were not affected by caffeine users and nonusers. Heart rates for the placebo subjects were significantly lower than all of the caffeine and ephedrine treatments groups, and there was no difference in the heart rates of the users and nonusers. RPE was lower for subjects that consumed the caffeine and ephedrine. The lower RPE suggested a psychological benefit from the caffeine-ephedrine supplement. The low perception of the amount of work that subjects performed may help to extend the amount of time to fatigue.

In another study, Drs. Bell and Jacobs (1999) found that a combination of caffeine and ephedrine significantly improved male subjects' time to exhaustion when compared with male subjects who consumed a placebo. The researchers used nine fit male subjects, who ingested a capsule containing either the placebo or the combination of caffeine plus ephedrine. Afterward, each subject completed the six Canadian Forces Warrior Tests. (The Warrior Test (WT) is a standard test that all land forces combat soldiers must perform within 22 minutes.)

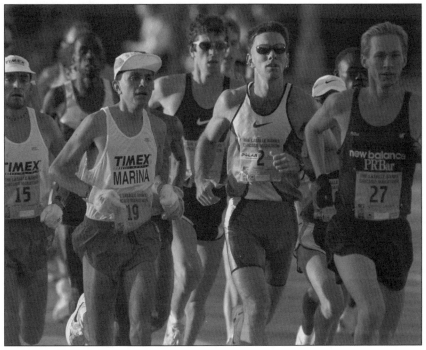

© Human Kinetics

The primary finding in this study was that the caffeine and ephedrine significantly improved the running times of the WT. Caffeine and ephedrine enabled the subjects to exercise at a higher percentage of the maximal aerobic power for a longer period of time when compared with the placebo trials. The faster performance time of the WT also correlated with a higher HR during the caffeine and ephedrine trial. These observations suggest that the improved performance may have been due to the CNS stimulatory effects of both caffeine and ephedrine. The data also suggest that the relationship between the perception of effort and heart rate response appears to have changed as a result of the ingestion of caffeine and ephedrine.

Although caffeine and ephedrine have been shown to be an effective ergogenic aid, there are aspects of this combination that bring caution to researchers. Dr. Bell and colleagues (1999) studied the combination of caffeine and ephedrine and its effects on body temperature. Caffeine and ephedrine have been shown to raise metabolic heat production, as well as body temperature. The effects of this combination on the body during a cold period are positive; during heat stress, it could be detrimental. It was concluded, however, that caffeine and ephedrine treatment was not detrimental to body temperature regulation while exercising in a hot, dry environment. Heat loss was greater in the caffeine and ephedrine treatments, and there was a trend for sweat rate to be increased. It is unlikely that heat storage and an increase in temperature would limit exercise performance.

Another factor to consider with caffeine and ephedrine supplementation is that the negative side effects are more likely to surface with noncaffeine users. Dr. Bell and colleagues (2000) performed an experiment using different dosages to test such side effects. With a reduction of caffeine and ephedrine, there was less chance of severe nausea or vomiting after ingesting the treatment. The lower dosage levels resulted in similar ergogenic effects as the higher dosages, which suggests that nonusers can benefit equally from the aid but with a lower dose and fewer side effects.

When you consider the results of these studies, you may note that the effects of caffeine and ephedrine on performance have not yet been fully explained. Differences in the subjects and methodology may account for these contradictory results. Further conflicting data may be attributed to the treatment duration, dosage, and specific combination of caffeine and ephedrine. Influences of caffeine and ephedrine are also dependent upon the health status of the subject, diet, exercise, and the interaction with other drugs (Sinclair and Geinger 2000). Finally, individual differences in athletic training status or aerobic capacity levels may be important variables that affect the body's response to caffeine and ephedrine.

Guidelines for Use

The studies seem to concur that an ergogenic benefit from caffeine can be achieved with a dose of 3 mg/kg (1.4 mg/lb) body weight. A dose of 5 to 6 mg/kg (2.3 to 2.7 mg/lb) body weight may be more effective at increasing free fatty acid levels. Therefore, to assure an ergogenic effect, we recommend a dose of 5 to 6 mg/kg body weight (about 460 to 540 mg for a 200-lb person) may be warranted. For the combination of caffeine and ephedrine, the effective dose appears to be 4 mg/kg (1.8 mg/lb) caffeine and 0.8 mg/kg (0.37 mg/lb) ephedrine. Thus, for a 150-lb person, that would be about 273 mg caffeine and 55 mg ephedrine.

Precautions

Caffeine isn't without potential side effects or problems, especially for athletes. The International Olympic Committee lists caffeine as a banned substance. While some amount of caffeine is allowed because of its occurrence in foods, a urinary level that exceeds 12 µg/ml will result in a doping violation and possible disqualification or suspension. The exact level of caffeine that appears in the urine varies with age, sex, weight, and metabolic rate. Table 3.1 lists various products that will result in doping violations if consumed in a large enough quantity.

Table 3.1 Examples of Caffeine-Containing Products That Might Exceed the Legal Limit

Caffeinated products	Amount to exceed limit
Brewed coffee	8 cups
Cola-type soft drink	17 cans
NoDoz	8 tablets
Excedrin	12 tablets
Chocolate	133 bars*

Limits set by the International Olympic Committee. * = 1.0-1.5 oz (23-43 g)

Adapted, by permission, from M.H. Williams, 1998, *The Ergogenics Edge*, (Champaign, IL: Human Kinetics), 153.

Caffeine is also considered a diuretic. Some people believe that caffeine may result in dehydration, which compromises thermoregulation caused by an increase in urine production and a decrease in plasma volume. A number of studies, however, have reported that caffeine ingestion before and during exercise does not alter urine volume or hydration status (Daniels et al. 1998; Dunagan, Greenleaf, and Cisar 1998; Falk et al. 1990; Wemple et al. 1997). In addition, these studies reported that core temperature was unaffected by caffeine ingestion, even at a dose of 10 mg/kg (4.5 mg/lb) body weight.

Another potential negative side effect associated with caffeine ingestion is the rise in blood pressure. For those who are mildly hypertensive, caffeine consumption can significantly increase heart rate and blood pressure at rest and during exercise (Daniels et al. 1998; Sung et al. 1995). Therefore, people with mild hypertension should avoid the use of caffeine before and during exercise.

Ephedra/ephedrine has a long history of safe use at the recommended amounts. Abuse of ephedrine—especially as a recreational drug—can lead to amphetamine-like side effects, including elevated blood pressure, rapid heart beat, nervousness, irritability, headache, urination disturbances, vomiting, muscle disturbances, insomnia, dry mouth, heart palpitations, and even death caused by heart failure (Blumenthal et al. 1998).

One study has shown that a single dose of ephedra caused mild elevation of heart rate but did not consistently affect blood pressure in otherwise healthy adults (White et al. 1997). But when taken at higher levels, ephedrine can cause drastic increases in blood pressure, as well as cardiac arrhythmias. Ephedrine is considered potentially habituating although it is unclear if the whole herb ephedra is likely to do the same thing (Blumenthal et al. 1998). Long-term overdose of ephedra or ephedrine (months or more) can also potentially cause kidney stones composed of ephedrine, though this condition is rare (Powell et al. 1998).

Anyone with high blood pressure, a heart condition, diabetes, glaucoma, hyperthyroidism, anxiety or restlessness, impaired circulation to the brain, benign prostatic hyperplasia with residual urine accumulation, pheochromocytoma, and those taking monoamine-oxidase–inhibiting antidepressants, digitoxin, or guanethidine should consult with a physician before using any type of product containing ephedra (Blumenthal et al. 1998). Ephedra-based products should be avoided during pregnancy and lactation, and they should be used with caution in children under the age of six years.

Certain medications may interact with ephedra. It is recommended that you discuss the use of ephedra and your current medication(s) with your doctor or pharmacist. In fact, before using an ephedra-based supplement, you should heed the warning listed on the product. For example, the following warning is contained on several ephedra-containing products currently on the market:

EPHEDRA WARNING

ONLY FOR USE BY ADULTS 18 YEARS OF AGE AND OLDER. DO NOT EXCEED *90 mg of ephedra alkaloids* (from the combination of all sources) per day - it will not improve results.
WARNING: Do not use if pregnant or nursing. If you have, or have a family history of, heart disease, thyroid disease, diabetes, high blood pressure, recurrent headaches, depression or other psychiatric condition, glaucoma, difficulty urinating, prostate enlargement, or seizure disorder, consult a health care provider before using this product. Do not use if you are using monoamine oxidase inhibitors (MAOI) or for two weeks after stopping an MAOI drug; certain drugs for depression, psychiatric or emotional conditions; drugs for Parkinson's disease; methyldopa; or any product containing ephedrine, pseudoephedrine, or phenylpropanolamine (ingredients found in allergy, asthma, cough/cold, and weight control products). Stop use and call a health care professional immediately if dizziness, severe headache, rapid and/or irregular heartbeat, chest pain, shortness of breath, nausea, noticeable changes in behavior, or loss of consciousness occur. Discontinue use at least two weeks prior to surgery. Do not take this product if you are allergic to pollen, bees, or bee products. Exceeding recommended dosage, or consuming product with caffeine, may cause serious adverse health effects, including heart attack and stroke. The maximum recommended dosage of ephedra alkaloids for a healthy adult human is no more than 100 mg in a 24-hour period for not more than 12 weeks. After the initial 12 weeks, consult your health care professional prior to resuming another 12-week regimen. **KEEP OUT OF THE REACH OF CHILDREN.**

Note: Ephedra use is banned by most sport governing bodies (e.g., International Olypmic Committee).

Carbohydrate

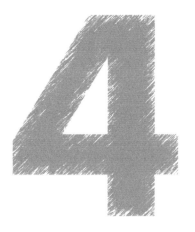

What Is It?

Carbohydrates are substances such as sugars, glycogen, starches, dextrins, and celluloses, and they are composed of the molecules carbon, oxygen, and hydrogen. As the primary macronutrient (fat and protein are the other two), carbohydrates are broken down and stored as glycogen in the liver and skeletal muscle. Once ingested, they also help sustain normal plasma glucose concentrations.

How Does It Work?

Because carbohydrates serve as the primary fuel source for endurance exercise, it makes sense that the consumption of this nutrient can enhance performance under specific circumstances (i.e., during prolonged endurance exercise). Research shows that the provision of exogenous carbohydrate during prolonged exercise can improve performance. This effect is potentially significant in events such as the marathon, in which competitors run 26.2 miles.

The Evidence: Pro or Con?

There is a huge volume of information regarding the administration of carbohydrates and its effect on exercise performance. Because of the volume, we will break down the research into the following three categories: pre-exercise, during exercise, and postexercise feeding. Furthermore, we'll examine the role of the glycemic index (GI) and the effects of carbohydrate loading on performance.

Pre-Exercise Feeding

Many studies have illustrated that pre-exercise ingestion of carbohydrates improves performance. One such study demonstrated that the ingestion of a one-liter sport drink an hour before a 15 K run followed by a 1.6 K performance run improved performance more so than water alone (Millard-Stafford et al. 1994). In another study with similar results, researchers found that ingesting a carbohydrate solution before and during intermittent, high-intensity shuttle running improved performance better than water alone (Nicholas et al. 1996).

In a more recent investigation (Febbraio et al. 2000a), scientists looked at the effect of carbohydrate ingestion before and during exercise. They took seven endurance-trained men and had them cycle for two hours at roughly 63% of their peak power output followed by a time trial (set at a workload of 7 kJ per kg [3.2kJ per lb] body weight). The study had four phases. During phase 1, subjects received a placebo beverage 30 minutes before exercise and at 15-minute intervals during exercise. In phase 2, subjects received a placebo beverage 30 minutes before exercise and a carbohydrate (CHO) beverage during exercise (2 g/kg body weight, or 0.9 g/lb; 6.4% solution). In phase 3, subjects received a CHO solution 30 minutes before exercise (2 g/kg body weight; 25.7% solution) and a placebo during exercise. Finally, during phase 4, subjects received a CHO solution 30 minutes before exercise (2 g/kg body weight; 25.7% solution) and a CHO solution (2 g/kg body weight; 6.4% solution) during exercise.

What happened? The time trials improved the most in phases 3 and 4. What this means is that the best way to improve performance is to consume carbohydrates before and during exercise. Even if you don't like consuming a meal or supplement before exercising, it would seem that consuming carbohydrates during exercise is paramount.

Furthermore, a study of carbohydrate use in the U.S. national field hockey team also showed positive results (Kreider et al. 1995). Seven members of the team were administered a carbohydrate drink containing 1 g/kg body weight (about 0.45 g/lb) four times per day while seven other team members ingested a placebo for seven days of intense training. Results indicated that the carbohydrate-supplemented group had a greater total energy intake, carbohydrate intake, and change (pre vs. post) in time to maximal exhaustion following training; moreover, they reported lower post-practice psychological fatigue.

These results by no means suggest that all research shows effects of pre-exercise carbohydrate feedings. For instance, Burke et al. (1998) had six well-trained cyclists consume carbohydrate in doses of 2 g/kg (0.9 g/lb) body weight. Two hours before exercise, subjects consumed carbohydrates that were high glycemic index (GI) (e.g., potato), low GI (e.g., pasta), or as a control, a low-energy jelly (meaning low-calorie). Subjects also consumed 10 g/100 ml glucose solution (total of 24 ml/kg body weight, about 11 ml/lb) before and during exercise. The exercise consisted of two hours of cycling at 70% $\dot{V}O_2$max followed by a performance ride at 300 kJ. The researchers found no difference in performance between groups.

Although it might seem that carbohydrate consumption has no significant effect on performance, that's far from the truth. What it does suggest is that if you eat carbohydrates during exercise, it may not matter what you eat before exercise (see next section).

Feeding During Exercise

The importance of consuming carbohydrates during exercise is more clearly demonstrated. In a double-blind, counterbalanced study, scientists examined 14 trained cyclists who participated in an 80-mile (self-paced) ride on two separate occasions during a simulated time trial. The trials were preceded by a prescribed diet with a final feeding three to four hours before exercise. Every 10 miles, subjects ingested either a noncaloric placebo or a carbohydrate maltodextrin supplement (5% maltodextrin and 2% fructose) at a dosage of 0.25 g/kg (0.11 g/lb) body weight (mean intake rate total of 37 g/hour, or 148 g total). The carbohydrate-supplemented group's finish times were 5% faster (241 vs. 253 minutes) than the placebo group's finish times. Riders who consumed the carbohydrate supplement were able to sustain higher intensities during the ride (Langenfeld et al. 1994).

In another study (Yaspelkis et al. 1993), seven well-trained male cyclists exercised at either 45 or 75% $\dot{V}O_2$max while receiving a placebo, 10% liquid carbohydrate supplement (18 g, three times an hour), or a solid carbohydrate supplement (25 g, two times per hour). During the first set, subjects cycled for 124 minutes, then rode a second set for 190 minutes, which was followed by a ride to exhaustion at 80% $\dot{V}O_2$max. Plasma glucose and insulin responses were significantly higher in the liquid carbohydrate trial when compared with the placebo trial. The time to exhaustion for the liquid (233.4 minutes) and solid carbohydrate (223.9 minutes) trials did not differ significantly, yet both were significantly greater than the placebo (202.4 minutes). In this case, it may not matter what kind of carbohydrate (solid vs. liquid) you ingest, but it clearly is better than no carbohydrates.

When you examine the scientific data in general, it becomes clear that consuming carbohydrates during exercise is a win-win proposition. Carbohydrate ingestion results in an increase in blood glucose, thus making this important fuel available for exercising muscles. In other words, when athletes consume carbohydrates, the ingested fuel promotes glucose uptake by muscles, which spares the liver from breaking down its own stores. This "saved" liver glycogen can then be used later in an exercise bout. Some evidence even indicates that consuming carbohydrates *during* exercise may spare muscle glycogen.

Keep in mind that the ingestion of carbohydrates during exercise will decrease the amount of fat that is used during exercise. That is a good thing if you're interested in maximizing performance! But if you're interested in just burning fat (and losing weight), then consuming carbohydrates during exercise may not be in your best interest.

Postexercise Feeding

Though eating carbohydrates is sacrosanct with many endurance athletes, it is our scientific opinion that in postexercise nutrition, the high-carbohydrate approach may not be ideal. In this case, a carbohydrate-protein (with a touch of fat) mixture may be best. Here's why.

Regarding the use of a carbohydrate-only meal versus a carbohydrate-protein mixture as a way to replenish skeletal muscle glycogen concentrations, there are several key points to consider. The preponderance of data does show that the addition of protein to carbohydrates generally has no further effect on glycogen repletion (Tarnopolsky et al. 1997; Van Hall, Shirreffs, and Calbet 2000). In fact, at a certain level of carbohydrate consumption (approximately 1.0 to 1.5 g/kg [0.45 to 0.68 g/lb] body weight every two hours postexercise), it is not likely that adding any more protein or carbohydrate has any further impact on the rate of glycogen repletion.

To illustrate this aspect, a recent paper by Rotman et al. (2000) compared a carbohydrate solution (1.7 g CHO/kg body weight, about 0.77 g/lb) with an isocaloric solution (i.e., having the same caloric content) of carbohydrate (1.2 g CHO/kg or 0.55 g CHO/lb) plus protein (0.5 g protein/kg or 0.23 g protein/lb). After approximately 1.5 hours of cycling, they consumed the solution immediately after and two hours postexercise. They found no difference in glycogen resynthesis.

You may think that adding protein is a waste; it doesn't help glycogen replenishment. You're right, but then again, you may be barking up the wrong tree. First of all, it indicates that there is a level of carbohydrate consumption that is sufficient to meet the needs of glycogen repletion.

Let's say that this level is 1.2 g/kg body weight (0.55 g/lb), which is about 84 g for a 154-lb athlete (or about 336 kcal carbohydrate), and let's presume that this amount has to be taken immediately and two hours after exercise. As you know, consuming 336 kcal carbohydrate is fairly easy. So why go overboard? Instead, add protein and a touch of fat (preferably unsaturated).

Does the added protein help in other ways? Absolutely. For instance, a recent study from the *Journal of Exercise Physiology* (Niles et al. 2001) found that ingesting carbohydrate (112 g) plus protein (40.7 g) improved running time to exhaustion more so than carbohydrate alone (152.7 g). Subjects had previously been glycogen depleted, and they consumed the drinks before the exercise test. In this case, the carbohydrate-protein combination may have allowed subjects to recover more quickly and perform better during a test of aerobic power.

More important, from a recovery point of view, the added protein is needed to help repair damaged muscle fibers. Work from Levenhagen et al. (2001) showed that a combination of carbohydrate, protein, and fat (10 g, 8 g, and 3 g respectively) significantly enhanced muscle protein synthesis. Work from the University of Texas at Galveston (Rasmussen et al. 2000) has also shown that the ingestion of essential amino acids postexercise will augment muscle protein synthesis.

So glycogen repletion is only one small part of the recovery equation. Repairing skeletal muscle is another, perhaps more important aspect. Athletes, primarily those in endurance sports, need to be aware that carbohydrates are not the end-all and be-all of required nutrients.

The bottom line: Unless you're an ultramarathoner, triathlete, or an athlete of that caliber, it is probably not necessary to ingest huge volumes of carbohydrates. If you're a recreational exercise buff, moderate carbohydrate with protein and fat will likely meet the needs of glycogen replenishment and the repair of skeletal muscle.

Glycemic Index: Does It Matter?

Well, yes and no. The health issues are intriguing. It may matter regarding long-term health and whether you consume a pre-exercise carbohydrate supplement before endurance exercise. For instance, a high GI diet may promote obesity. Pawlak and colleagues (2001) found that rats became fatter on high glycemic-index starch diets than rats on lower GI diets. In addition to the obesity factor, the GI also affects the appetite after a high GI meal. Ludwig et al. (1999) demonstrated that voluntary energy intake after a high GI meal was 53% greater than after a medium GI meal and 81% greater than after a low GI meal. The implication: You can control your appetite better after a low GI meal, which therefore positively affects body composition.

With regard to the possible application during exercise, scientists found that a low glycemic meal before incremental exercise on a bike (200 watts until exhaustion) resulted in lower plasma lactate levels (lactic acid) versus a high glycemic meal (Stannard et al. 2000). These results suggest that for high-intensity exercise, a low GI meal before training may allow you to train harder. Kirwan, O'Gorman, and Evans (1998) support this notion by illustrating that a moderate GI meal (versus a high GI meal) resulted in an exercise time to exhaustion that was 16% longer (using a semirecumbent bike exercise).

Not all studies show an effect of glycemic index, however. For instance, Australian scientists compared pre-exercise, high and low GI meals (30 minutes before exercise) and found no differences in cycling performance (Febbraio et al. 2000b).

Carbohydrate Loading: Does It Work?

Perhaps the best study to examine the effects of carbohydrate loading was performed by a group of Australian scientists (Burke et al. 2000). In this crossover design study, seven well-trained cyclists performed a 100 K time trial three days after carbohydrate loading—ingesting 9 g/kg (4.1 g/lb) body weight daily—or after ingesting carbohydrates at 6 g/kg (2.7 g/lb) body weight daily (the placebo). The subjects consumed a carbohydrate breakfast two hours before the time trial, and they consumed 1 g/kg (0.45 g/lb) body weight per hour in the form of a drink during exercise. During the time trial, there were four 4 K sprints and five 1 K sprints. Muscle glycogen concentrations were significantly increased with carbohydrate loading; however, muscle glycogen utilization, time to complete the trial, and mean power output were not significantly different between the carbohydrate-loading and placebo group. Does this suggest that carbohydrate loading doesn't work?

Perhaps what it does show is that if you consume carbohydrates during endurance exercise, it may not matter if you carbohydrate load before the exercise or not. Nor will it matter what you consume before exercise. This study also raises the possibility that carbohydrate loading helps via a placebo effect. Alternatively, it may help from the standpoint of higher pre-exercise liver glycogen stores that could delay the onset of hypoglycemia during prolonged exercise. Bottom line: Carbohydrate ingestion during exercise is paramount. Whether you carbohydrate load or not, it doesn't change the fact that you need to consume carbohydrates during exercise to improve performance.

Guidelines for Use

Before you go on a carbohydrate-consuming rampage (as many endurance athletes do), keep in mind that the amount of carbohydrates you consume may not be a critical issue. Unless you're going to embark on exercise that is continuous in nature and lasts longer than at least 1.5 hours, be on the safe side and moderate your carbohydrate consumption. And remember: It certainly does not hurt to consume carbohydrate during exercise; in fact, it probably helps.

Also, be aware that each person has particular likes and dislikes when it comes to carbohydrate consumption. You must tailor these needs specifically; there is no one-size-fits-all prescription.

Pre-Exercise

Perhaps for shorter duration events (e.g., 5 K, 10 K runs), the ingestion of a high GI carbohydrate 5 to 10 minutes before the event might be beneficial. Alternatively, the consumption of a low GI carbohydrate 30 to 60 minutes before an endurance event may be beneficial as well.

During Exercise

Ingesting carbohydrates (30 to 60 g/hour) during exercise will improve performance. Similarly, if you consume approximately one liter or so of

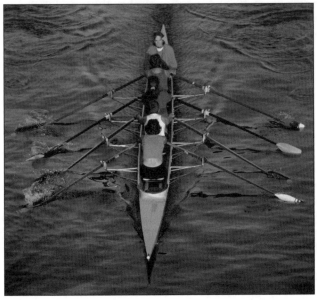

© PhotoDisc

water per hour of exercise (preferably more in a hot environment) with these carbohydrates, this supplement will help alleviate the dehydration-induced decrease in performance. According to McArdle, Katch, and Katch (1999), "Carbohydrate feeding during exercise at 60-80% of aerobic capacity postpones fatigue by 15 to 30 minutes (general range of improvement between 15 and 35%)."

Postexercise

Unless you're a marathon or ultramarathon-type athlete, the consumption of roughly 1.0 to 1.5 g carbohydrate per kg body weight (0.45 to 0.68 g/lb) immediately postexercise and one hour postexercise may be sufficient to meet the needs of glycogen replenishment—that is, of course, if you eat regular mixed meals (carbohydrate, protein, fat) throughout the day. Furthermore, we would even suggest adding protein to those postexercise meals—about 0.5 g protein per kg body weight (0.23 g/lb). This protein provides the needed amino acids for skeletal muscle repair and recovery. You don't need a degree in mathematics to decipher these recommendations: Just remember, as a general rule of thumb, to consume roughly twice as many carbohydrate calories as protein.

If you train at extremely high levels (e.g., if you're a Tour de France cyclist or ultramarathoner), it may be necessary to increase your carbohydrate intake to high levels (10 to 12 g/kg body weight daily; about 4.55 to 5.45 g/lb). Keep in mind that some people have difficulty consuming that many calories in the form of carbohydrates; thus, it may be wise to consume additional fat. There is increasing evidence that high-fat diets do not hurt performance and may actually improve performance (see chapter 10, "Fat").

Carbohydrate Loading

Again, this technique applies only to those who compete or participate in long-duration activities (two hours or more). Whether it works or is needed is not completely known. However, if your diet is chronically high in carbohydrates, then you are depleting your muscles after a prolonged bout of exercise and repleting them every time you consume a high-carbohydrate, postworkout meal. Further, consuming carbohydrates during exercise may offset any effect of carbohydrate loading.

Note: Two excellent resources on sports nutrition and exercise science can be found at www.sportsci.org. Dr. Louise Burke, from the Australian Institute of Sport, provides easy-to-read, practical advice on carbohydrate needs for sport (see figure 4.1). Another fine resource is *Nutrition for Health, Fitness, and Sport* by Dr. Melvin Williams.

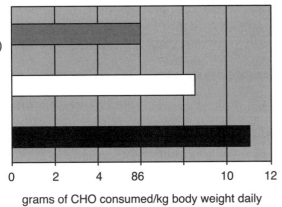

Figure 4.1 Carbohydrate intake goals. Modified from L. Burke, www.sportsci.org/news/compeat/grams.html.

Galactose: A Superior Sugar?

Although the majority of research on sugar replacement during exercise has focused on sucrose, glucose, fructose, or some combination thereof, some interesting data suggest that galactose may possess better ergogenic properties. Galactose is a simple monosaccharide that isn't stored in your body to any significant extent. If you compared the chemical structure of galactose to glucose, they are nearly identical except for the position of one hydroxyl (OH) group. Unlike glucose, however, galactose does not elicit a large insulin response; it maintains an even level of plasma glucose and insulin. Where can you find galactose? One place is milk, where the milk sugar lactose is broken down into glucose and galactose. But even if you're lactose intolerant, you can still consume galactose without any untoward effects.

So why the hoopla over galactose? In a study presented at the Experimental Biology meeting in Orlando, Florida (King, Cooke, and O'Hara 2001), scientists compared the effects of galactose with other sugars. Five well-trained cyclists performed an exercise test 30 minutes after drinking one liter of one of the following supplements: sucrose/glucose, fructose/glucose polymer, galactose, or galactose/polymer. The exercise test consisted of a bicycle ride 90% $\dot{V}O_2$max for 50 minutes followed by 10 90-second repetitions with a 180-second recovery at 55% $\dot{V}O_2$max. They found that the subjects who consumed the galactose or galactose/polymer-containing drinks lasted on average 4% longer on the bicycle than the sucrose/glucose group and 31% longer than the fructose/glucose group. While these results demonstrate some strong evidence in favor of galactose, future research on galactose as an endurance ergogenic aid should shed more conclusive light on this interesting sugar.

Precautions

Each person needs to determine which carbohydrate works best for him or her. Generally, glucose, sucrose, and maltodextrins have similar effects when ingested during exercise. Although fructose (in high doses) may cause gastrointestinal upset, small amounts of it may help promote the absorption of glucose when consumed simultaneously.

Carnitine

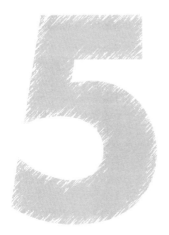

What Is It?

Carnitine is a compound that helps transport long-chain fatty acids into the mitochondria of the cell, where fat can be used as fuel. Carnitine (or L-carnitine, to be exact) is obtained from your diet—primarily in meat and dairy products. It can also be made from the amino acids lysine and methionine in chemical reactions that require vitamin C. Other forms of carnitine include the DL-form, which should be avoided (see "Precautions" section).

How Does It Work?

The amount of glycogen stored in skeletal muscles has a direct effect on one's performance in an endurance event. If you're glycogen depleted, your performance can suffer. The ingestion of L-carnitine has been speculated to spare skeletal muscle glycogen by enhancing fatty acid oxidation (using fat for energy). By sparing the use of glycogen during the initial stages of prolonged endurance exercise (via the increased utilization of free fatty acids), L-carnitine may allow your body to tap into your muscle glycogen reserves later in a race or performance. Therefore, this glycogen-sparing effect (via L-carnitine) may aid endurance performance. Furthermore, this chain of events has led to the suggestion that carnitine is an effective fat-loss dietary aid.

The Evidence: Pro or Con?

There have been several investigations on the effects of carnitine on fat oxidation and exercise performance. To say the least, the evidence is mixed; nonetheless, some data support a beneficial effect of carnitine supplementation.

In a study done by Italian researchers (Vecchiet et al. 1990), 10 moderately trained young men were used to determine the effects of L-carnitine. The study was a double-blind, placebo-controlled, crossover trial, which means that each subject received the placebo and the carnitine treatment. (In essence, they served as their own control.) One hour before exercise, they consumed (orally) 2 g L-carnitine. Afterward, they commenced a bike exercise in which the workload increased by 50 watts every three minutes until the subjects reached exhaustion.

The results? The carnitine-supplemented trials showed an increase in $\dot{V}O_2$max and total work performed (see figures 5.1 and 5.2).

Similarly, Marconi et al. (1985) found that carnitine loading (4 g/day orally for two weeks) increased $\dot{V}O_2$max by 6% (54.5 to 57.8 ml/kg/min) in long-distance, competitive walkers. Additionally, taking 2 g L-carnitine daily for 28 days resulted in an increase in fat oxidation during cycling exercise at an intensity of 66% of $\dot{V}O_2$max (Gorostiaga, Maurer, and Eclache 1989). Research from the Institute of Sports Medicine in Turin, Italy, similarly found an increased fat oxidation during treadmill exercise (Wyss et al. 1990).

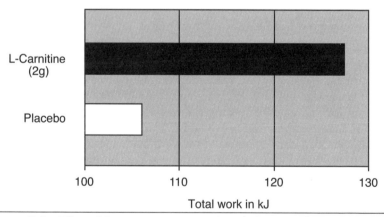

Figure 5.1 Effect of 2 g L-carnitine on total work (kJ). Data from Vecchiet et al. 1990.

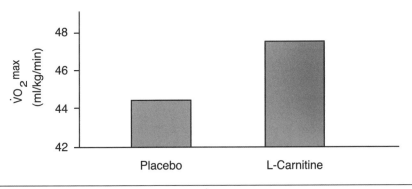

Figure 5.2   Effect of 2 g L-carnitine on $\dot{V}O_2$max. Data from Vecchiet et al. 1990.

While the previous data show promise for L-carnitine as an effective supplement, not all studies show ergogenic effects of acute and chronic L-carnitine supplementation. According to French researchers, "In normal human subjects the increased demand for fatty acid oxidation resulting from exercise seems to be adequately supported by endogenous levels of carnitine" (Oyono-Enguelle et al. 1988). Noted sport nutrition researcher Matt Vukovich, PhD, of South Dakota State University found that one and two weeks of carnitine supplementation (6 g daily) neither changes muscle carnitine content nor increases fat oxidation (Vukovich, Costill, and Fink 1994). Studies by Greig et al. (1987) and Colombani et al. (1996) have also found no effect of acute carnitine consumption (2 g) or chronic consumption (2 g daily for two to four weeks) on endurance exercise performance.

An interesting side note about carnitine is the data regarding its use in clinical situations. For instance, one study looked at 41 patients experiencing cardiac insufficiency. They were given either a placebo or L-carnitine (1 g, three times per day for 120 days). According to these researchers, "A significant improvement in performance (significantly higher maximum performance during bicycle ergometry) could be found within the carnitine group on the 60th and 120th day of L-carnitine supplementation" (Loster et al. 1999). Additionally, supplementation with 2 g L-carnitine daily for three months improved exercise performance during a stress test. In patients with chronic stable angina, supplementation with L-carnitine increased endurance from 7.8 minutes to 8.6 minutes—a 10% improvement (Iyer et al. 2000). The mechanism(s) for this effect is unclear, and though carnitine may help those with cardiac problems, it still isn't known if this applies to endurance athletes.

Guidelines for Use

The logical question is whether carnitine supplementation is worthwhile. For every study that shows a positive effect, there is a similar one that shows no effect. If it's any consolation for those who use carnitine, at least it doesn't have an ergoglytic effect; that is, it doesn't decrease exercise performance. So for those who wish to use it, a few recommendations are in order.

Carnitine supplementation may help you only if you consume gram doses. In other words, consuming 2 g carnitine one hour before exercise might impart a beneficial effect. Perhaps taking 2 g daily for a period of several weeks may even have ergogenic effects. Because of biological variability and the fact that we each have unique responses to different supplements or drugs, we do believe it would be a bit parochial to presume that carnitine supplementation is useless for everyone. It might help a few of you, whereas for others, it may be a waste of time and money.

Precautions

Oral L-carnitine consumption is safe, but if you choose to use it, don't use DL-carnitine. Just use L-carnitine. DL-carnitine can't be used by your body. In fact, Japanese researchers (Watanabe et al. 1995) found that 900 mg/day L-carnitine versus DL-carnitine showed that "L-carnitine increases and DL-carnitine decreases exercise tolerance in patients with impaired exercise tolerance (i.e., cardiac disease)."

Coenzyme Q10

6

What Is It?

Coenzyme Q10 (CoQ10), also known as ubiquinone, is one of a series of molecules that are involved in the production of adenosine triphosphate (ATP). CoQ10 is also known as a strong antioxidant, which controls the damaging effects of free radicals (the compounds that cause cellular damage during metabolism). You can find CoQ10 naturally in your body's cell membranes and as part of the mitochondria, the "powerhouse" of the cell.

How Does It Work?

CoQ10 aids in the production of energy (ATP) by transporting the electrons within the mitochondria. Because of its involvement in making ATP and its role as an antioxidant, some scientists have theorized that by taking extra CoQ10, endurance athletes may be able to enhance aerobic exercise performance as well as combat the damage caused by exercise-induced free radical generation.

The Evidence: Pro or Con?

For those with heart problems, CoQ10 may actually help improve exercise tolerance or capacity. In one study (Kamikawa et al. 1985), 12 patients (aged 56) with stable angina pectoris were administered 150 mg CoQ10 per day for four weeks. (Angina pectoris is characterized by severe pain and a feeling of constriction in the chest [heart] area, and it is typically caused by a deficient oxygen supply to the heart muscle.) Exercise time improved to 406 seconds in the CoQ10-treated group compared with 345 seconds in the placebo-treated group. Although 60 seconds may not seem relevant, it is a statistically significant difference. In other words, the CoQ10 significantly affected the subjects who ingested it. Additionally, the average CoQ10 plasma concentration increased from 0.95 to 2.20 mcg per ml after CoQ10 treatment. According to these researchers, "CoQ10 is a safe and promising treatment for angina pectoris."

In a study from the University of Tsukuba in Japan, researchers tested the effects of CoQ10 administration on rats with muscle injury (Shimomura et al. 1991). They compared CoQ10-treated rats versus placebo-treated rats after 90 minutes of downhill running. After the exercise bout, they found that the CoQ10-treated rats had lower levels of blood creatine kinase and also of lactate dehydrogenase enzymes, which are indirect markers of muscle damage. These scientists believed that "coenzyme Q10 treatment protected skeletal muscles against injury caused during exercise, but not against damage related to the inflammatory processes after exercise."

So the question becomes this: What happens if you give CoQ10 to healthy athletes? A study from the Vuokatti Sports Testcenter in Finland revealed some interesting findings (Ylikoski et al. 1997). They used 25 elite, national-level cross-country skiers as subjects and put them on a six-week supplementation period of either a placebo or 90 mg CoQ10 per day. Because the study design was a crossover study, every subject underwent both the placebo and CoQ10 treatments. In essence, they served as their own control group. Blood levels of CoQ10 increased from 0.8 to 2.8 mcg per ml. $\dot{V}O_2$max did not change (-0.6% to 0.1%) in the placebo group but improved by 2.1 to 3.9% in the CoQ10-treated group. Whether this increase in aerobic power necessarily translates into an improvement during an actual athletic event is unknown at this time. Subjectively, "94% of athletes felt that CoQ10 supplementation was beneficial: 72% noted a clear positive effect and 22% a slight benefit in their exercise performance and their recovery time" (see figure 6.1).

Despite these positive findings, the majority of studies on CoQ10 supplementation in healthy people have failed to find an ergogenic effect. For instance, Braun et al. (1991) took 10 male bicycle racers and had them perform a graded exercise test on a bicycle before and after eight weeks of CoQ10 supplementation (100 mg per day). Although the CoQ10 supplemented group experienced a significant rise in blood levels of CoQ10 versus the placebo group, they found no differences in cycling performance, $\dot{V}O_2$max, submaximal physiological parameters, or lipid peroxidation. In other words, CoQ10 didn't do a thing.

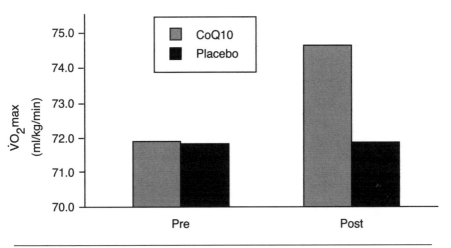

Figure 6.1 Maximal oxygen uptake. Data from Ylikoski et al. 1997.

In another study, Weston et al. (1997) examined the effects of CoQ10 supplementation on male cyclists and triathletes (1 mg/kg or 0.45 mg/lb body weight daily for 28 days). Even though blood CoQ10 levels increased significantly in the supplemented group, there was "no consistently significant effect on oxygen uptake, anaerobic and respiratory compensation thresholds, blood lactate, glucose and triglyceride kinetics, heart rate, blood pressure during and after graded cycling to exhaustion." Again, CoQ10 failed to perform as an ergogenic aid.

Another study (Snider et al. 1992) found no effect of CoQ10 supplementation in male triathletes. In two other studies, CoQ10 showed to be largely ineffectual in middle-aged trained men (Bonetti et al. 2000) and middle-aged untrained men (Porter et al. 1995).

For athletes, CoQ10 probably has no ergogenic effect. Its role as an antioxidant, however, merits further study, and this reason may be a convincing one for athletes who choose to use it as a supplement.

Guidelines for Use

For a few endurance athletes, supplementing with 90 to 100 mg CoQ10 daily may impart an ergogenic effect, but the majority of data do not support such an effect. Nevertheless, its antioxidant properties may be of value to athletes. Additionally, those suffering from congestive heart failure, irregular heartbeat, or angina may experience improved function as a result of supplementation.

Precautions

There are no known side of effects of CoQ10 supplementation in healthy adults; however, its effect on pregnant and breastfeeding women is unclear. For instance, in one study, Noia et al. (1996) found that as plasma CoQ10 levels increased, the contractile activity of the uterine muscles also increased. Further studies are needed to elucidate the significance of these findings. Until more research is done, women who are pregnant or breastfeeding may want to avoid supplementing with CoQ10.

Colostrum

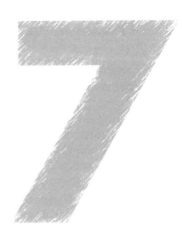

What Is It?

Milk is a great source of protein and other healthy nutrients, such as calcium and vitamin D. It is also, of course, our first nourishment in the first days of life. However, in the first 24 to 72 hours, when we undergo a period of rapid development, we are actually supported by a special type of mother's milk called colostrum. It is the first mammary secretion provided for newborns, and it occurs just before the onset of genuine lactation.

The formulation of colostrum is much more complex than that of simple milk; its components are not found in such high concentrations anywhere else in nature (Kishikawa et al. 1996; Kuhne et al. 2000). There are several major components to colostrum, two of which are currently undergoing vigorous investigation: The growth factor fraction (IGF-1) and the immunoglobulin fraction. A third remaining fraction contains enzymes, proteins, assorted peptides, and other compounds of interest to athletes (Mero 1997; Pakkanen and Aalto 1997).

How Does It Work?

There is evidence to suggest that the IGF-1 in colostrum stimulates cellular (muscle) growth (Kishikawa et al. 1996; Kuhne et al. 2000). The current hypothesis is that the combination of high-quality proteins and IGF-1 found in colostrum may optimally stimulate muscle protein synthesis (Buckley et al. 2001).

In addition to its anabolic effects on skeletal muscle, IGF-1 may have metabolic effects that could improve muscular endurance. Endurance training often leads the body to an enhanced ability to utilize fats as energy during exercise. This increase in fat utilization may lead to increased glycogen sparing, which may ultimately improve endurance performance.

For example, IGF-1 has been shown to stimulate lipoprotein lipase (LPL) activity—that is, it breaks down fat for energy—and it may also inhibit insulin activity in fat cells (Kern et al. 1989). The combination of an increase in LPL activity and a reduction in insulin activity may enhance fat metabolism. This chain of events leads to an increase in free fatty acid levels in the blood and thus is used for energy. Theoretically, colostrum supplementation enhances the effects of endurance training through the actions of IGF-1 on LPL and skeletal muscle.

The Evidence: Pro or Con?

In a double-blind, placebo-controlled study—neither athletes nor researchers knew who was getting colostrum or placebo—39 fit young men (ages 18-35) completed an eight-week running program, running three times a week for 45 minutes per session (Buckley et al. 1998). They consumed either a placebo (whey protein) or 60 g colostrum per day. At the start, and again at the fourth and eighth week, all subjects did two treadmill runs to exhaustion, with 20 minutes' rest between runs. At the beginning of the study, no differences existed in treadmill running performance. At week four, both groups had improved similarly in treadmill running performance; however, at week eight, the colostrum group ran significantly farther and did more work than the placebo group during the treadmill test (see figures 7.1 and 7.2).

Furthermore, the colostrum-supplemented group showed a trend toward reduced serum creatine kinase levels. Creatine kinase is a critically important muscle-cell enzyme, which some experts believe can be used as a marker of muscle-cell damage. If blood creatine-kinase concentrations rocket upward, it's often a sign that significant muscle damage has occurred. On the other hand, if creatine kinase levels stay fairly normal, some researchers believe that the person has not experienced much muscle trauma (Buckley et al. 1998).

Guideline for Use

The research is intriguing, but more studies are still needed to validate efficacy for endurance athletes. The current research suggests a

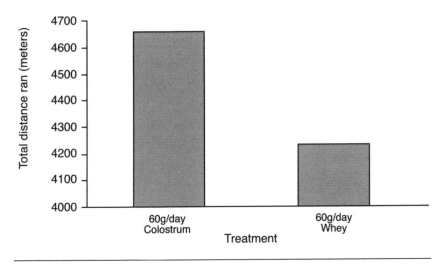

Figure 7.1 Effect of colostrum versus whey supplementation on total distance run. Data from Buckley et al. 1998.

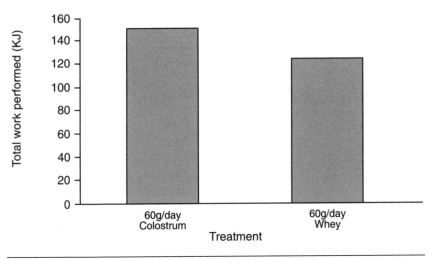

Figure 7.2 Effect of colostrum versus whey supplementation on total work completed. Data from Buckley et al. 1998.

recommended dose of 60 g/day. However, we would surmise that a lower dose of colostrum (perhaps 20 g), combined with a high-quality protein (such as whey), may offer better benefits to the endurance athlete. Future research should examine this possibility.

Precautions

Colostrum contains a wide range of growth promoting factors. One could argue that it has an effect on doping-related testing. However, a study was performed in which human growth hormone, IGF-1 levels, and hematocrit were measured in the blood before and after four weeks of supplementation (60 g/day) (Kuipers 2001). The results demonstrated that none of the parameters changed, and the doping test was negative.

Creatine

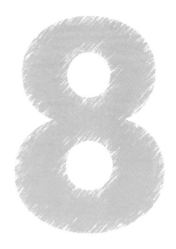

What Is It?

Creatine (Cr) is a nitrogenous organic compound (see figure 8.1) that is synthesized to a small extent (2%) in the liver, pancreas, and kidneys from the amino acids arginine, methionine, and glycine (Pearson et al. 1999). Approximately 95% of all the creatine stores in the body are found in skeletal muscle. Creatine can also be obtained through exogenous sources, such as foods that are high in protein like fish and beef (see table 8.1 for creatine content in select foods) (Williams, Kreider, and Branch 1999).

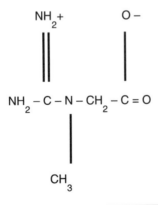

Figure 8.1 Molecular structure of creatine.

Table 8.1 Creatine Content in Select Food

Food	grams Cr/lb	grams Cr/kg
Cod	1.4	3.0
Beef	2.0	4.5
Herring	3.0-4.5	6.5-10.0
Milk	0.05	0.1
Pork	2.3	5.0
Salmon	2.0	4.5
Shrimp	Trace	Trace
Tuna	1.8	4.0

Creatine Content in Select Food. Adapted, by permission, from M.H. Williams, M.R. Kreider, and D. Branch, 1999, *Creatine: The power supplement* (Champaign, IL: Human Kinetics), 15.

How Does It Work?

The human body relies on three main metabolic systems for energy—either by direct means from the adenosine triphosphate–phosphocreatine (ATP-PCr) system, or indirectly through aerobic and anaerobic glycolysis. The ATP-PCr system is always the first to respond to exercise, and it provides immediate energy. A drawback, though, to the quick energy and accessibility of phosphocreatine, or creatine phosphate (PCr), is its rapid depletion (Gilliam et al. 2000). The depletion of the PCr stores occurs at an extremely high rate (less than 15 seconds) (Edwards et al. 2000). Decreased synthesis of energy (ATP) brought about the notion that creatine supplementation may be a means of increasing PCr and creatine stores, thus reducing fatigue and increasing performance (Pearson et al. 1999).

To demonstrate this theory, Dr. Demant (Demant and Rhodes 1999) reported that Cr supplementation of 20 to 30 g/day for three days or longer is believed to enhance exercise performance in two ways. First, by increasing the initial amounts of PCr in the muscle, Cr may provide a greater initial source of energy. Second, providing more free Cr aids the regeneration rate of PCr during recovery.

Recently, it has been theorized that increasing muscle PCr levels by creatine supplementation may also improve high intensity endurance events (90 seconds to four minutes). PCr supplementation would decrease the reliance on anaerobic glycolysis, and it would reduce lactate accumulation. The onset of fatigue would thus be delayed (Prevost, Nelson, and Morris 1997; Stout et al. 2000; Volek and Kraemer 1996).

The Evidence: Pro or Con?

Dr. Harris and colleagues (1993) conducted one of the earliest studies on high-intensity endurance performance with creatine supplementation. Using well-trained distance runners as subjects, the researchers demonstrated that oral creatine supplementation improved cumulative, repeated running times following four 300-m sprints by 1.5 seconds and four 1000-m runs by 13.0 seconds. Individual running times for the final measured repeat run times improved as well: Final 300-m running time decreased by 0.7 seconds, and 1000-m running time decreased by 5.5 seconds.

One criticism of this study, however, is that all subjects were asked to run at 90 to 95% of their maximal effort. Each running pace was therefore dictated by the subjective opinion of each runner. Although a threat to the study's internal validity, these are intriguing findings because traditionally, the primary contribution of PCr to ATP maintenance takes place within approximately the first 10 seconds of intense physical exercise.

How, then, can creatine aid endurance performance if its utility comes during the first 10 seconds? It may be a combination of reasons: One, PCr may aid ATP resynthesis for up to three minutes, albeit in a decreasing role with time and intensity of work (Bangsbo et al. 1990); two, it may also act as an energy shuttle between the mitochondria and muscle fibers, which suggests that creatine may help produce ATP aerobically (Bessman 1986, 1987; Wallimann et al. 1992). If this scenario evolves into fact through more research, then creatine may very well enhance endurance performance.

In an early study to test this very question, Dr. Balsom and colleagues (1993) investigated the effects of creatine supplementation on endurance exercise performance. In a double-blind study, 18 moderately active to well-trained male subjects were evenly divided into treatment and placebo groups. After completing a standard $\dot{V}O_2$max test (a measure of aerobic fitness), each subject performed the following pre- and post-test runs, respectively: A treadmill run to exhaustion at 120% of $\dot{V}O_2$max designed to elicit fatigue between three and six minutes, and a terrain run of approximately 6 K on a forest track. After six days of creatine supplementation, no significant differences in time to exhaustion, terrain runs, or $\dot{V}O_2$max were noted between groups. It was thus concluded that creatine supplementation had no effect on endurance performance.

Other reports, however, of anaerobic running performance suggest that creatine may or may not improve exhaustive work bouts that last between 40 and 240 seconds. A study by Dr. Earnest and colleagues (Earnest, Almada, and Mitchell 1997) sought to determine if creatine supplementation would improve intermediate-length, anaerobic treadmill running. In a double-blind, placebo-controlled trial, 11 male subjects received a creatine or glucose placebo at 20 g/day for four days and 10 g/day for six days. After two weeks of rehearsal, subjects performed two exhaustive runs, separated by eight minutes of recovery, at individually prescribed intensities. Time to exhaustion for independent runs, for both runs combined (total time to exhaustion), and blood–lactic acid concentration were examined for each run. Running times in the creatine group were negligible for the first run (1.5 seconds), improved more during the second run (3.2 seconds), and were significantly greater for total time to exhaustion (4.7 seconds).

In a follow-up to this investigation, Dr. Smith and colleagues (1998) examined the effect of creatine ingestion on time to exhaustion. They used intense cycle ergometry exercise bouts to establish the estimates of anaerobic capacity and critical power (the measure of maximal aerobic power). Fifteen (eight male and seven female) recreationally active university students were selected for this study. The results demonstrated a significant effect for creatine on anaerobic capacity by 12.9% but with no change in critical power.

Recently, Dr. Jacobs (Jacobs, Bleue, and Goodman 1997) and Dr. Prevost (Prevost, Nelson, and Morris 1997) demonstrated significant increases in time to exhaustion during intense cycle ergometry with creatine supplementation. After creatine loading, physically active men and women improved their endurance capacity by 24% and 8%, respectively. Dr. Prevost and colleagues (1997) hypothesized that creatine loading increased exercise capacity and diminished the exercise-induced rise in plasma lactate levels by delaying anaerobic glycolysis. Anaerobic glycolysis produces lactate, which leads to muscle fatigue. Therefore, by delaying anaerobic glycolysis, you may delay muscle fatigue. In contrast to these findings, Dr. Febbraio and colleagues (1995) demonstrated no significant differences in time to exhaustion and intramuscular lactate levels during cycle ergometry at 115 to 120% of $\dot{V}O_2$max.

Despite the studies done on anaerobic exercise bouts, few studies have been conducted to determine the effects of creatine supplementation on submaximal endurance exercise performance. In one study, Dr. Nelson and colleagues (2000) reported that creatine loading in male and female athletes resulted in a 12% increase in the anaerobic threshold as well as a decrease in blood lactate during incremental cycle tests. In agreement, Dr. Stout and colleagues (2000) demonstrated that creatine supplementation in highly trained female athletes delayed the onset of neuromuscular fatigue (similar to anaerobic threshold) by 13% (see figure 8.2). Dr. Stout's study appears to support the hypothesis proposed by Dr. Prevost and col-

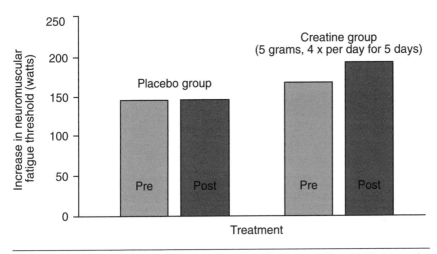

Figure 8.2 Creatine's effects on neuromuscular fatigue threshold. Note the significant change in the creatine group (p < 0.05). Data from Stout et al. 2000.

leagues (1997) and Drs. Volek and Kraemer (1996). They suggested that increasing muscle creatine phosphate levels by creatine supplementation may decrease the reliance on anaerobic glycolysis and reduce intramuscular lactate accumulation, which, therefore, delays the onset of fatigue.

Guidelines for Use

More research is needed on to the effect of creatine and endurance exercise. It appears that creatine may help cycling performance but may hinder running performance (which would be due primarily to the additional body weight). To increase creatine and PCr levels in skeletal muscle, athletes should utilize a loading phase for one week: 20 g/day (four doses of 5 g each) for five to seven days. A maintenance dose of 2.5 to 5 g/day should be enough to maintain skeletal muscle creatine and PCr levels.

Precautions

Creatine supplementation has been studied in healthy populations for more than 10 years, and the only confirmed side effect has been weight gain. There are also anecdotal reports of stomach or gastrointestinal upset. Nonetheless, there is no scientific evidence to show that regular creatine supplementation is harmful to healthy adults.

Dimethylglycine

What Is It?

N, N, dimethylglycine, or dimethylglycine (DMG), is an extract from liver, seeds, and nuts. It was discovered in 1943 and marketed under the name *pangamic acid*, or vitamin B15. This substance was originally touted as a cure for various ailments such as cancer and glaucoma, but it is now the belief that supplementation with DMG could increase performance.

How Does It Work?

The various claims made by the marketers of DMG include improved utilization of oxygen and increased mental alertness. DMG supposedly increases tissue oxygen uptake and exercise performance (Stackpoole 1977), though most of these studies were criticized for their poor research design (Gray and Titlow 1982; Herbert 1979).

The Evidence: Pro or Con?

A study conducted by Dr. Pipes (1980) used 12 male track athletes (aged 18-21). The subjects received either 5 mg pangamic acid or a placebo for one week. Performance was measured by having the subjects run on a treadmill at a 7.5% incline at a speed of 9.0 mph. The speed was increased 1.5 mph every minute until exhaustion.

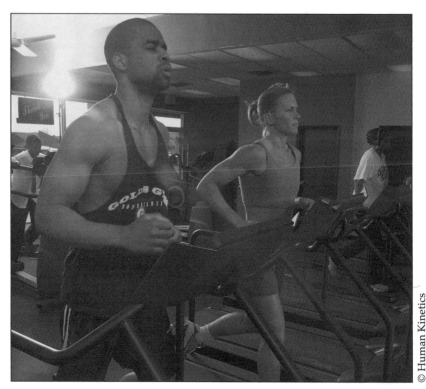

© Human Kinetics

The subjects receiving pangamic acid improved their running times significantly (23.6%) compared with the placebo group (0.9%), and there was a significant increase in $\dot{V}O_2$max (a measure of aerobic power) in the treatment group (27.5%) versus the placebo (3.3%). According to these data, pangamic acid seems to be an effective aid in improving performance. This conclusion had also been reached in an earlier study by Dr. Kemp (1959); however, neither one of these studies involved subject or investigator blinding.

In another study (this one, double-blind), the effect of pangamic acid on treadmill performance was determined using 16 male track athletes (Gray and Titlow 1982). The athletes ingested per day either six tablets pangamic acid (50 mg/tablet) or a placebo for three weeks. Before and after supplementation, the subjects performed a treadmill test to determine maximal heart rate, treadmill time to exhaustion, recovery heart rate (at minutes one and three), blood glucose levels, and lactate levels. The results showed no significant difference between groups for any of the parameters.

The ingestion of DMG also demonstrated no improvement for performance in a study conducted by Drs. Black and Sucec (1981). They had 18 physically active men perform an inclined treadmill test after the ingestion of either six tablets of calcium pangamate (50 mg/tablet, two per meal) or a placebo for two weeks. The results showed no significant improvement in $\dot{V}O_2$max or 15-minute running performance time.

Furthermore, a more recent study by Dr. Bishop and colleagues (1987) showed similar results. The study used 16 trained runners, who showed no significant improvement in $\dot{V}O_2$max, heart rate, or total run time when compared with a placebo. These results supported a similar study conducted by Dr. Girandola and colleagues (1980).

Guidelines for Use

DMG has been proposed to increase oxygen utilization via skeletal muscle, which should logically lead to an increase in endurance performance. But because DMG has not shown much potential as an endurance enhancement, we do not recommend that athletes supplement with this nutrient.

Precautions

Safety studies have been conducted on the effects of DMG using rabbit models (Reap and Lawson 1990). When testing for the immunomodulating capacity of DMG, no toxic or adverse side effects occurred. Additionally, when DMG (300-600 mg/day) was administered to human subjects for several days, no toxicity was noted (Gascon et al. 1989). Regardless, there are no data to support its use as an ergogenic aid.

Fat

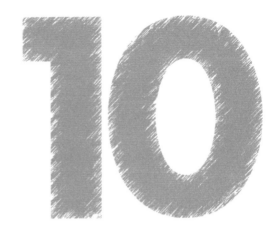

What Is It?

Fat (or lipids) is similar to carbohydrate in that they're made of carbon, oxygen, and hydrogen atoms. However, the ratio between hydrogen and oxygen in fat differs radically as compared with carbohydrates (fat has much more hydrogen). Nearly all of dietary fat (98%) exists as triglycerides (also known as triacylglycerol), which are glycerol molecules that are each connected to three fatty acid molecules.

It is important to note that different dietary fats exert different physiological effects. For instance, saturated fats may elevate blood cholesterol and perhaps increase one's risk of heart disease, whereas the unsaturated fats may actually offer *protection* from heart disease. Another type of fat is "trans" fat, which is found when polyunsaturated fat is partially hydrogenated (so that it can be solid at room temperature, such as with stick margarine or shortening). The consumption of trans fat may also increase one's risk for cardiovascular disease.

For an excellent review on this subject, see Hu, Manson, and Willett (2001) in the February issue of the *Journal of the American College of Nutrition*.

How Does It Work?

Fat and carbohydrate are the main fuels for exercise with fats more important at lower exercise intensities. Our bodies have a limited ability to store carbohydrates while we in essence have a "limitless" supply of fat. For instance, a person who is 154 lb and of average body composition (not obese) has about 2,000 kcal stored carbohydrates and approximately 140,000 kcal fat (70 times more energy). Comparing these numbers, you can clearly see why fat deserves reconsideration as an ergogenic aid. The question becomes, how does one take advantage of such a rich resource of energy?

There is valid scientific evidence that demonstrates that eating a higher fat diet does not necessarily compromise performance; in fact, it may help it. This does not, however, suggest that you "fat load" in the hopes of bringing your marathon time from three-and-a-half hours to three hours flat. But what is intriguing about the data on fat is that sports nutrition experts have routinely ignored it. Fat has received such a bad rap that we have whole categories of food that cater to the low-fat mentality. Many athletes may actually be consuming insufficient calories, and fat may just be the best way to ingest enough energy to meet the demands of endurance training and competition.

For an excellent review on fat intake for athletes, read the article by Drs. Brown and Cox (2001). They suggest that one of the more important metabolic adaptations to a high-fat diet is an increase in intramuscular fat stores. With added fat stores in muscle, endurance athletes have added fuel for exercise. This fat may then be oxidized (burned) at a higher rate and intensity than has been previously suggested.

The Evidence: Pro or Con?

First of all, we know that endurance-trained athletes oxidize proportionately more fat and less carbohydrate as compared with sedentary people. Whether we can take advantage of this physiological adaptation as a method to improve performance is debatable as the evidence regarding fat versus carbohydrate diets for endurance performance is far from resolved. Despite the lack of a final word, let's examine some of the existing literature in an attempt to glean some basic advice for the endurance-training athlete. We'll break up our analysis into two methods of fat consumption: acute feeding and chronic feeding.

Acute Feeding

What happens when you consume a high-fat meal versus a high-carbohydrate meal before exercising? Okano et al. (1996) compared the effects of a high-carbohydrate meal with a high-fat meal consumed by subjects four hours before cycling exercises. They used 10 endurance-trained collegiate males who consumed either a single high-carbohydrate meal (79% carbohydrate, 10% fat, 11% protein; 1,116 kcals) or a single high-fat meal (30% carbohydrate, 61% fat, 9%

protein; 1,126 kcals). They exercised at 65% of $\dot{V}O_2$max for the first 120 minutes, followed by an increased intensity (80% of $\dot{V}O_2$max) until exhaustion. They found no effect on exercise performance.

A study from the Oxford Lipid Metabolism Group in Oxford, England (Whitley et al. 1998) took eight well-trained cyclists ($\dot{V}O_2$max of 65 to 84 ml/kg/minute) and had them consume in grams per 70 kg (154 lb) body weight either a high-carbohydrate meal (215 g carbohydrate, 26 g protein, 3 g fat) or a high-fat meal (50 g carbohydrate, 14 g protein, 80 g fat). The cyclists exercised for 90 minutes at 70% of $\dot{V}O_2$max and followed up with a 10K time trial. The researchers found no differences in performance between the carbohydrate and fat groups.

Chronic Feeding

Although eating a single high-fat meal doesn't seem to have an ergogenic effect, the same cannot be said for chronic consumption of a high-fat diet. For instance, a study from New Zealand (Brown and Cox 2000) looked at 32 endurance-trained cyclists who for 12 weeks consumed either a high-fat diet (47% kcal from fat, 37% carbohydrate) or high-carbohydrate diet (14% fat, 69% carbohydrate). After 6 and 12 weeks on the diet, they performed 20 K road time trials. Researchers found no significant difference in performance between groups.

What is interesting about this study is not so much that eating a high-fat diet didn't affect performance but that eating a high-carbohydrate diet didn't necessarily help performance either. Does this mean we should re-examine the notion that endurance athletes should be on chronic high-carbohydrate diets? Perhaps it does.

In another study, Lambert et al. (1994) compared the effects of a high-fat diet (70% fat, 7% carbohydrate) with a high-carbohydrate diet (74% carbohydrate, 12% fat) on exercise performance in trained cyclists. After two weeks of being on the diets, subjects had to perform an exercise test of cycling to exhaustion at 85% of peak power and 50% of peak power output. When the subjects cycled at 85% of peak power, exercise time to exhaustion was not different between diets. However, when they were tested at the lower intensity (50% peak power), the high-fat group performed better.

In another study, scientists at the State University of New York (Muoio et al. 1994) compared three dietary interventions, each one lasting a week. The percentage of each macronutrient was as follows: normal diet (61% carbohydrate, 24% fat, 14% protein), high-fat diet (50%, 38%, 12%, respectively), or high-carbohydrate diet (73%, 15%, 12%). Running time to exhaustion and $\dot{V}O_2$max was greatest in the high-fat diet group as compared with the other two groups (see figures 10.1 and 10.2).

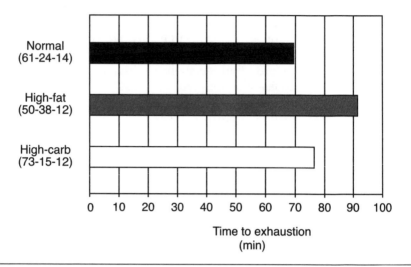

Figure 10.1 Time to exhaustion. Data from Muoio et al. 1994.

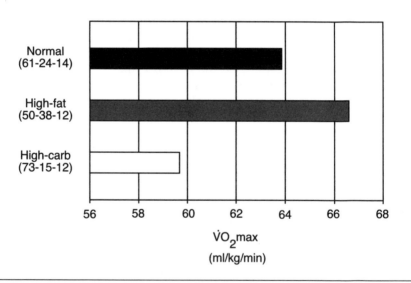

Figure 10.2 Effect of dietary fat on $\dot{V}O_2$max. Data from Muoio et al. 1994.

According to these investigators, "Increased availability of FFA (free fatty acids), consequent to a high-fat diet, may provide for enhanced oxidative potential as evidenced by an increase in VO_2max and running time. This implies that restriction of dietary fat may be detrimental to endurance performance." In other words, a higher-fat diet may not necessarily be as bad as we thought for the endurance athlete.

In recent study, Horvath et al. (2000) examined a longer period of dietary intervention (four weeks) and compared low (16%), medium (31%), and high (44%) fat diets in 12 male and 13 female runners (42 mi/week). All diets were designed to be isocaloric (i.e., have the same caloric content), but what Horvath et al. (2000) discovered was that runners on the low-fat diet consumed 19% fewer total calories than on the medium or high-fat diets. Also interesting was that over 50% of the runners were not willing to increase their fat intake to 44% of total caloric intake. We'd guess that many runners exhibit a fat phobia conditioned by years of negative information about fat. The results of the study indicated that endurance time improved by 14% in the medium versus the low-fat group. However, the highest fat group had lower lactate levels (39% less) after the endurance run.

This information illustrates a potential problem that endurance athletes may run into (no pun intended)—they may not be consuming enough calories! Although eating "low fat" has been a godsend to companies who make these products, it certainly is not the best way for runners and other endurance athletes to eat. Furthermore, a high-fat diet, providing adequate calories, does not compromise anaerobic power.

Of course, not every study shows an improvement when athletes consume more fat. Equally important is that performance is not diminished on a high-fat diet. According leading scientists, the duration in which you consume a high-fat diet is important (Brown and Cox 2001). A complete metabolic adaptation to a high-fat diet may take 6 to 20 weeks.

Another consideration is the type of fat consumed. It isn't known if certain fats (e.g., saturated versus polyunsaturated) are better regarding performance or if a particular ratio of fats is optimal. Certainly, more research needs to be performed in this area, though it is safe to say that a low-fat intake (10 to 15% fat) may be detrimental to endurance athletes (Pendergast, Leddy, and Venkatraman 2000).

Guidelines for Use

According to the existing research, eating a high-fat meal prior to exercise or competition does not help performance, and the consumption of a low-fat diet (10 to 15%) may actually hurt one's performance. One reason could be the fact that fat provides more than twice the calories per gram as carbohydrates or protein, and getting sufficient calories may be a problem for endurance athletes. The solution? Eat more fat.

Additionally, while many experts recommend eating a high-carbohydrate diet, it isn't clear that this strategy does not necessarily translate to a performance advantage. It is entirely possible that if you're an endurance athlete, such as a marathon runner who runs on average 50 to 100 miles per week, you may need to concentrate more on getting enough calories to provide fuel for exercise and promote a quick recovery. Eating more fat may just be the key.

As an estimate, let's say athletes need to consume roughly 50 kcal/kg body weight, or 23 kcal/lb (McArdle, Katch, and Katch 1999). For a 150-lb runner, that would be 3,450 kcal/day. So let's take the theoretical macronutrient ratio as shown in figure 10.3. Let's assume a 20% protein, 30% fat, and 50% carbohydrate diet (the higher end of carbohydrate intake), which would translate to 690 kcal protein (172 g), 1,035 kcal fat (115 g), and 1,725 kcal carbohydrate (431 g). Per lb body weight, the numbers would be 1.15 g protein, 0.77 g fat, and 2.87 g carbohydrate (per kg body weight: 2.5 g protein, 1.7 g fat, and 6.3 g carbohydrate).

With this theoretical model, the carbohydrate intake is slightly lower than the recommendations of Burke (www.sportsci.org/news/compeat/grams.html), and the protein intake is higher than the recommendations of Lemon et al. (1997). Does this represent the best dietary approach for endurance athletes? That's a difficult question to answer because each individual may respond differently to identical diets.

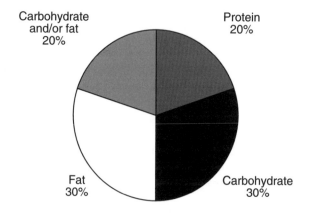

Figure 10.3 A theoretical macronutrient ratio for endurance athletes. Data from Pendergast, Leddy, and Venkatraman 2000.

One thing is clear, though: Eating a high-carbohydrate diet (70% kcal) is not ideal for everyone. At that high an intake, it sometimes becomes problematic just getting enough calories. Some would even argue that a protein intake of 2.5 g / kg (1.2 g / lb) body weight is excessive as well, which raises a couple of issues to consider: one, that such a high protein intake is not harmful (Poortmans and Dellalieux 2000); and second, the extra protein ingested could contribute to glycogen resynthesis. Perhaps one could lower the protein intake to 2 g per kg (0.9 g / lb) body weight and make up the remaining calories as fat and carbohydrates. Regardless, endurance athletes need to experiment with different macronutrient ratios to determine what works best for their particular training needs.

Precautions

Too much fat, too little fat. Both options have potentially harmful health consequences. First the issue of too much fat: We would tend to concur with the view held by Dr. Willett (1998) that "diets high in fat do not appear to be the primary cause of the high prevalence of excess body fat in our society, and reductions in fat will not be the solution." An intriguing article published in *Science*, which is considered the world's most prestigious scientific journal, debunks the notion held so dearly by mainstream nutritional science (Taubes 2001) that dietary fat is the culprit regarding a variety of diseases (e.g., heart disease, diabetes). We're told to eat less saturated fat and you'll live longer. How much longer? You'll be surprised.

According to the *Science* article, between 1987 and 1992, three independent investigations from groups of scientists came up with the same answer (interestingly, this kind of information rarely makes the mainstream press). Using computer models, they estimated that if only 10% of our calories came from saturated fat (as recommended; so total fat intake would be 30%), "a healthy non-smoker might add 3 days to 3 months." In other words, if you avoid saturated fat for your entire lifetime, instead of dying at age 65, you could expect to die at age 65 plus, on average, about two extra weeks. This isn't exactly a compelling reason to consume a low saturated fat diet for an entire lifetime. The most telling quotation from this article was from Dr. Willett: "They say you really need a high level of proof to change the recommendations, which is ironic, because they never had a high level of proof to set them."

How about eating too little fat? Well, clearly if you're eating less fat, you're probably eating more of something else, which usually means carbohydrates. Unless you're a bodybuilder or strength-power athlete, most individuals generally do not add pure protein as a substitute for fat. (How many runners do you see snacking on a can of tuna or on a piece of skinless chicken breast?) If you end up eating more carbohydrates (usually refined), this diet could cause a host of problems (e.g., increased triglycerides, decreased HDL, insulin resistance). For an endurance athlete, it may not matter because exercise alone would likely counteract the possible harm caused by a diet high in high glycemic-index carbohydrates.

In conclusion, whether you eat lots of fat or lots of carbohydrates may not matter too much if you exercise. But eating too little fat (10 to 15% of kcals) is definitely not the right approach and may ultimately hurt your performance.

Ginseng

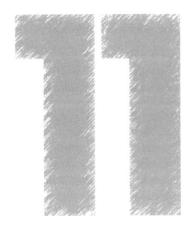

What Is It?

Ginseng is a popular herbal remedy traditionally used by the Chinese for thousands of years. There are several kinds of commercially available ginseng: American, Chinese, Japanese, Korean, and Siberian. A more descriptive examination of these different ginseng species can be found in an excellent review by Bahrke and Morgan (2000). For the purpose of this book, we will only refer to the general properties of ginseng.

How Does It Work?

The mechanism of action of this herb is still unclear; nonetheless, many studies have been conducted on ginseng's effect on the central nervous system, neuroendocrine function, carbohydrate and lipid metabolism, immune function, and the cardiovascular system. Most of the research, however, is highly contradictory, and one possible reason is that the ginsenoside content of the ginseng root can differ. Both the method of extraction and even the season in which the root is harvested can affect ginseng content (Gillis 1997).

One recent study has shown that treatment with ginseng during exercise significantly increased free fatty acid levels in plasma and maintained plasma glucose levels. Additionally, glycogen levels in the liver and skeletal muscle were slightly higher in the ginseng-supplemented group compared with the placebo group. This difference indicates that the use of ginseng may increase endurance performance by altering the body's choice of fuel—that is, free fatty acids used preferentially over glucose (Wang and Lee 1998).

The Evidence: Pro or Con?

In a double-blind, randomized, crossover study on ginseng (Pieralisi, Ripari, and Vecchiet 1991), 50 male sports teachers (aged 21-47) ingested either a placebo or a combination of ginseng extract, dimethylaminoethanol bitartrate, vitamins, minerals, and trace elements at a dose of two capsules per day for six weeks. Before and after supplementation, the subjects performed a treadmill test at an increasing workload to determine $\dot{V}O_2$max. The subjects who supplemented with ginseng significantly increased $\dot{V}O_2$max as compared with the placebo group. Additionally, the ingestion of a ginseng supplement resulted in a significant decrease in plasma lactate levels and heart rate during the exercise test. What is interesting is that the less fit subjects (those with lower $\dot{V}O_2$max) responded more significantly to ginseng supplementation than did the more fit subjects (those with higher $\dot{V}O_2$max). Thus, untrained subjects beginning an exercise program may benefit from ginseng more than highly trained athletes.

Contrary to these findings, studies conducted five years later on ginseng showed different results. In the first study, 36 men participated in a randomized, double-blind, placebo-controlled trial (the best study design possible) (Engels and Wirth 1997). These subjects ingested 200 or 400 mg ginseng per day for eight weeks. With 31 subjects completing the study, the results showed no significant changes in $\dot{V}O_2$max, blood lactic acid concentration, heart rate, or perceived exertion.

Another study done on ginseng also showed no improvement in endurance performance (Allen et al. 1998). Twenty young men and eight young women were given 200 mg ginseng per day for three weeks in a double-blind, randomized study. Before and after supplementation, subjects performed a graded exercise test on a Schwinn Airdyne cycle ergometer. No significant changes were reported between groups for $\dot{V}O_2$max, exercise time, workload, plasma lactate, heart rate, and rate of perceived exertion at all workloads.

Supporting the previous two studies mentioned, Dr. Ziemba and colleagues (1999) conducted a more recent study that demonstrated no ergogenic effects of ginseng. Fifteen soccer players (mean age of 19 years) were randomly assigned to receive either 350 mg ginseng per day or a placebo for six weeks. Before and after treatment, the subjects performed an incremental bicycle ergometer test with the workload increasing until exhaus-

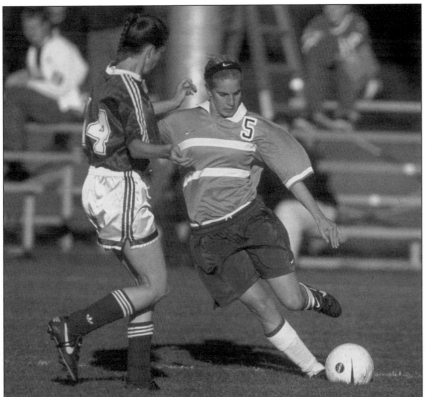

© Human Kinetics

tion. There were no significant improvements in either group for $\dot{V}O_2max$ or lactate threshold.

These studies demonstrate that it isn't clear whether ginseng supplementation acts as a useful ergogenic aid. Because there are different types of ginseng, it is necessary that more research be done to parcel out differences (if they exist) among the various forms.

Guidelines for Use

Early studies with animal models showed some potential with the use of ginseng; however, most of the studies using human subjects have not shown similar potential. As we mentioned, perhaps the data on ginseng are tainted because of the different species of ginseng or the various percent concentrations of the active ingredient. More research definitely needs to be done before definitive recommendations can be made.

Precautions

Long-term administration of ginseng has not shown any toxicity (Aphale et al. 1998). A study by Dr. Scaglione and colleagues (1996) was conducted to determine the safety and efficacy of ginseng extract. The researchers had 227 subjects ingest 100 mg ginseng for 12 weeks, and laboratory values for 24 safety parameters showed no significant differences from pre- to postvalues. All ginseng currently sold over the counter in the United States is generally considered a safe herbal supplement.

Glutamine

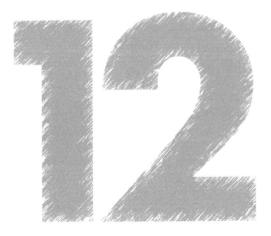

What Is It?

Glutamine is usually defined as a nonessential amino acid; you don't need to consume it to have a healthy diet. However, it should be considered a *conditionally* essential amino acid because during times of stress, the body's need for glutamine may not be met by the normal endogenous (within the body) synthesis of this important amino acid.

It's interesting to note that glutamine, not carbohydrates or fat, is the preferred fuel source for rapidly dividing cells such as enterocytes (intestinal cells) and lymphocytes (your immune system cells). Glutamine also has a role as a nitrogen carrier for acid-base balance (pH balance) and as a precursor for important macromolecules, such as proteins and nucleic acids.

As mentioned, glutamine may have a protein-sparing effect during times of severe stress. According to a recent article published in the *World Journal of Surgery*, "Most naturally occurring food proteins contain 4 to 8% of their amino acid residues as glutamine; therefore less than 10 g of dietary glutamine is likely to be consumed daily by the average person. In contrast to this usual dietary availability, studies in stressed patients indicate that considerably larger amounts of glutamine (20-40 g/day) may be necessary to maintain glutamine homeostasis" (Labow and Souba 2000). Whether prolonged endurance training induces a stress similar to surgery is debatable; however, there is evidence that suggests a potential utility to glutamine supplementation.

How Does It Work?

Glutamine is the most abundant amino acid in plasma and in skeletal muscle; it accounts for greater than 60% of the total intramuscular free amino acid pool (Lacey and Wilmore 1990; Rowbottom, Keast, and Morton 1996). Skeletal muscle and adipose tissue are sites of glutamine synthesis (Frayn et al. 1991) as are the lungs, liver, and brain. Because the body has a considerable capacity to make glutamine, scientists have always assumed that you don't need extra glutamine in your diet.

This assumption is now becoming suspect, though, because this amino acid becomes depleted during times of severe stress, such as infection or injury. The body may react to prolonged exercise and overtraining as a stressful event; that is, extensive training may lead to a significant drop in blood levels of glutamine. Therefore, whether or not glutamine supplementation is necessary or effective is a worthwhile question to investigate.

Another factor in this issue is that glutamine is also a favored fuel source by the gastrointestinal tract. Thus, one might theorize that by providing extra exogenous glutamine (via dietary supplementation), you can spare intramuscular glutamine while feeding the gastrointestinal tract. And sparing muscle glutamine is important. Maintaining normal levels of intramuscular glutamine is vital in preventing the breakdown of skeletal muscle protein (Antonio and Street 1999).

In addition to the gastrointestinal tract, other parts of the body (such as cells of the immune system, kidneys, and hair follicles) use this amino acid as fuel. In the liver, glutamine is used for glucose and urea synthesis, whereas the brain utilizes glutamine as a precursor for neurotransmitter substances. Obviously, glutamine has a wide variety of roles, but more research needs to be done to understand its impact on exercising individuals.

The Evidence: Pro or Con?

We do know that glutamine may have a protein-sparing, or anti-catabolic, effect. For instance, a study done at the Nestle Research Center in Switzerland compared the effects of different diets on rats treated with a hormone (dexamethasone) that causes muscle wasting (glucocorticoids) (Boza et al. 2001). Rats received a diet that consisted of either casein, mixed whey proteins (with or without glutamine), or carob protein plus essential amino acids. They found that the dexamethasone treatment of these rats reduced weight gain, muscle glutamine, and muscle and intestinal protein synthetic rate. Interestingly, only when glutamine was added as a free form

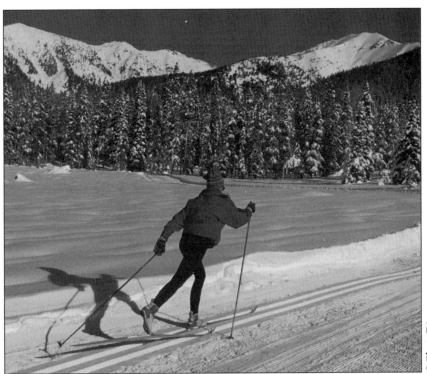

© PhotoDisc

amino acid did muscle protein synthesis improve (from 16 to 24%). According to the authors, "We speculate that glutamine provided in dietary protein is extensively metabolized by the splanchnic tissues and does not influence peripheral glutamine status to the same extent as glutamine provided in a free amino acid form."

So does this mean that taking free form glutamine might prevent the loss of muscle mass in humans who partake in extensive exercise training? Is there a minimal amount of muscle mass that endurance athletes should have, and could this muscle mass be spared by taking supplemental glutamine? Nobody knows for certain the answers to these questions.

In terms of muscle mass, we do know that endurance athletes are among the leanest and smallest of athletes. Perhaps the one area where glutamine may be helpful to athletes is via its effect on the immune system. Athletes that exercise excessively or are overtrained may be immunosuppressed, so glutamine ingestion may help alleviate illness. An improved immune system would avert the loss of training days, which would indirectly affect performance.

In a 1998 study, Castell and Newsholme demonstrated another indirect effect of glutamine: "Oral glutamine, compared to placebo, appeared to have a beneficial effect on the incidence of infections reported by runners after a marathon." For instance, in a study of athletes who had consumed either a placebo or glutamine immediately after and two hours after running (marathon or ultramarathon) or rowing training, it was found that those who consumed glutamine reported fewer infections than the placebo group (see figure 12.1) (Castell, Poortmans, and Newsholme 1996). The levels of infection were lowest in the middle-distance runners and highest in runners after a marathon or ultramarathon and in the elite rowers after training.

In conclusion, supplemental glutamine may not directly affect performance of the endurance athlete. If it can alleviate or prevent illness caused by intense training or competition, then an athlete who supplements with it would be less likely to miss training days and therefore receive an indirect benefit.

Guidelines for Use

One may be able to get adequate glutamine via the ingestion of dietary protein because most protein foods are composed of 4 to 8% glutamine. By eating an additional serving of protein (e.g., fish, chicken, eggs), one should be able to maintain adequate levels of glutamine.

Regarding supplementation, different doses elicit different biological responses: A minimum of 2 g glutamine is needed to elicit an increase in

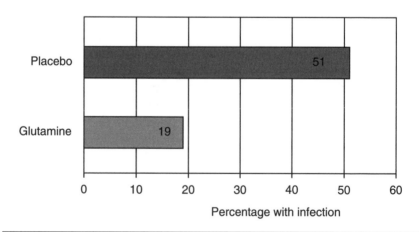

Figure 12.1 Percentage of athletes reporting infection after glutamine consumption.

plasma growth hormone levels; an 8 g dose is effective in promoting glycogen resynthesis; and doses as high as 80 g (for a 200-lb person) seem to indicate an anti-catabolic effect for those who exercise regularly. But 80 g glutamine is probably not feasible for most athletes interested in using this amino acid.

According to studies done with hospital patients, doses needed to alter protein balance favorably are quite substantial, 0.2 to 0.6 g/kg body weight daily (approximately 0.1 to 0.3 g/lb body weight, or 20 to 60 g for a 200-lb individual). In other words, an effective working dose could potentially be 10% of one's body weight (in grams).

It should also be recognized that glutamine supplementation need not be cycled; that is, one should not alternate between off and on periods of use. Because glutamine may be intimately involved in the recovery process, the consumption of it as part of a postexercise meal is important.

Precautions

Studies from Ziegler et al. (1990) have shown that short- and long-term glutamine supplementation is safe in humans. Oral doses of glutamine— 0.1 to 0.3 g/kg body weight, or approximately 0.05 to 0.13 g/lb body weight—produce an acute rise in plasma glutamine as well as amino acids known to be end products of glutamine metabolism (alanine, citrulline, arginine). However, there was no evidence of toxicity as demonstrated by no change in ammonia or glutamate levels. As a component of total parenteral nutrition, glutamine supplementation has been shown to be a safe and effective anti-proteolytic agent (it prevents muscle breakdown). A glutamine dose that appears to be a safe option for endurance athletes is 0.285 to 0.570 g/kg body weight (0.13 to 0.26 g/lb body weight; 26 to 52 g for a 200-lb person).

Glycerol

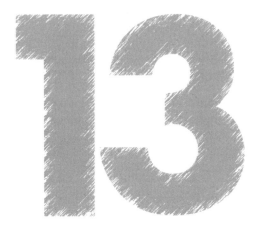

What Is It?

Also known as glycerin, glycerine, or 1,2,3-propanetriol, glycerol is a "colorless, odorless, sweet-tasting, syrupy liquid . . . a trihydric alcohol" (www.bartleby.com/65/gl/glycerol.html). You can find glycerol in various products such as protein bars, and it is there to improve the taste, sweetness, and palatability of the bar. Of course, it also provides dietary energy. Glycerol has 4.32 calories per gram, so its energy content is similar to that of protein and carbohydrates.

But what makes glycerol such an anomaly is how it is classified. Should it be classified as a protein? No. A carbohydrate? Actually, not that either. Glycerol doesn't fit the structural definition of a carbohydrate. Carbohydrates are polyhydroxy aldehydes or ketones, and glycerol is classified as a polyhydroxy alcohol ($C_3H_8O_3$).

When you consume glycerol, it doesn't produce significant increases in plasma (blood) insulin or glucose. However, when you *ingest* glycerol, it triggers an entirely different chain of events. First, it may be incorporated into triglycerides and phospholipids, which are structural components of cell membranes; then, it is burned directly for energy and ultimately used by the liver and kidneys to make glucose.

Again, ingested glycerol is not structurally a carbohydrate nor does it behave similarly to "traditional" carbohydrates such as glucose, sucrose, or starches. Glycerol is what is called, according to Hunt and Groff (1990), a "noncarbohydrate source." They write, "When dietary intake of carbohydrate is reduced and blood glucose concentration declines, a hormonal triggering of accelerated glucose synthesis from noncarbohydrate sources occurs. Lactate, pyruvate, glycerol (a catabolic product of triglycerides), and certain amino acids represent important noncarbohydrate sources."

How Does It Work?

Because glycerol acts as a sponge to soak up additional water, researchers theorize that glycerol can act as an ergogenic aid vis-à-vis its hyperhydrating properties (Wagner 1999). Scientists aren't sure exactly how glycerol does this, but they have proposed several theories. Some scientists believe that glycerol is reabsorbed by the kidneys, which in turn leads to more water being reabsorbed by the body (Wagner 1999). Another theory states that glycerol increases what is called *plasma osmolality*, which is an increase in the concentration of dissolved substances in blood. An increase in plasma osmolality then causes anti-diuretic hormone (ADH) to decrease less (which typically decreases when you hyperhydrate yourself), and all of this ultimately results in an increased urinary excretion.

Nonetheless, we'll let scientists parse the mechanisms of glycerol action. The more important question is whether it can actually help exercise performance.

The Evidence: Pro or Con?

As with much of science, there is evidence that shows glycerol to be an effective ergogenic aid, and there are data that show a neutral effect. In other words, it either helps or has no effect.

In one study (Lyons et al. 1990), four men and two women took a placebo or a dose of glycerol, 1 g/kg body weight mixed with 3.3 ml orange juice per kg body weight plus 21.4 ml water per kg body weight (0.45 g/lb glycerol, 1.5 ml/lb orange juice, and 9.73 ml/lb water). The researchers then had them exercise at 42°C at 25% relative humidity for 90 minutes on a treadmill at 60% of their maximal oxygen uptake (2.5 hours after ingestion). They found that urine volume decreased before exercise, sweat rate increased, and rectal temperature was lower during exercise. These findings suggest that glycerol ingestion was helpful in maintaining normal body temperature during exercise in the heat.

A study from the *International Journal of Sports Medicine* (Montner et al. 1996) also showed glycerol to have an ergogenic effect. These investigators performed two double-blind, placebo-controlled, crossover studies. In the first study (see figure 13.1), they gave 11 fit adults glycerol (1.2 g/kg [0.54 g/lb] glycerol in 26 ml/kg [11.8 ml/lb] body weight solution) or a placebo (26 ml/kg [11.8 ml/lb] body weight aspartame-flavored solution) one hour before cycle exercise to exhaustion at 60% of maximum workload

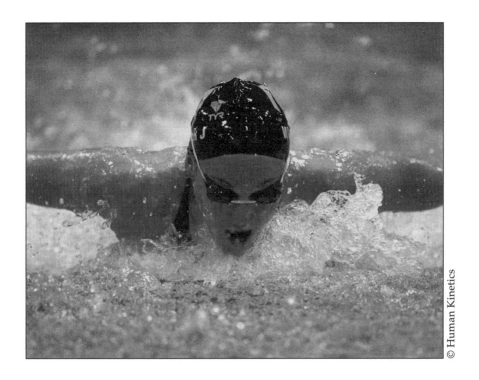

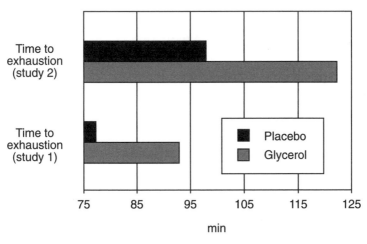

Figure 13.1 Effect of pre-exercise glycerol supplementation on endurance performance. Data from Montner et al. 1996.

(temperature 23.5-24.5ºC, humidity 25-27%). When subjects took glycerol, the average heart rate was 2.8 bpm lower and endurance time was 21% longer.

In the second study, they determined whether the same pre-exercise regimen followed by a carbohydrate oral replacement solution (ORS) during exercise had any further effect. They found, again, that when glycerol had been taken, endurance time was 25% longer. Interestingly, body temperature (measured rectally) did not differ between placebo or glycerol.

Not all studies have shown an ergogenic effect of glycerol consumption. For instance, Murray et al. (1991) had five women and four men consume various beverages during cycling exercise for 90 minutes at 50% of $\dot{V}O_2$max in 30°C at 45% relative humidity. Beverages tested included 10% glycerol solution (G), a 6% carbohydrate-electrolyte beverage (CE), 6% carbohydrate-electrolyte beverage with 4% glycerol (CEG), and a water placebo (WP). Subjects ingested the beverages at regular intervals during the first 60 minutes of exercise. Each subject went through each treatment in a counterbalanced order. In short, these investigators found that "these data indicate that there are no substantial metabolic, hormonal, cardiovascular, or thermoregulatory advantages to the consumption of solutions containing 4% or 10% glycerol during exercise."

To conclude, glycerol consumption either has a neutral effect, or it may in fact help endurance performance and thermoregulation. In a review, Wagner (1999) goes into exquisite detail about how glycerol may (or may not) affect performance.

Guidelines for Use

Although glycerol does not work for everyone, individual responses vary and one may find that doing a case study might reveal glycerol to have a positive ergogenic effect. If you do choose to use it, a glycerol solution containing 1 g glycerol per kg (0.45 g glycerol/lb) body weight should be ingested one to two hours before endurance exercise. To make dosing simple, glycerol-containing drinks are commercially available, which athletes can use. Heed the following warning though, if you decide to invest time into this supplement: "As with any sport drink or nutritional aid, if an athlete decides to try glycerol-induced hyperhydration, he or she should experiment with it in training before using it in competition" (Wagner 1999).

Precautions

Glycerol is well tolerated and safe at an oral dose of 1 g/kg body weight (about 0.45 g/lb, or 90 g for a 200-lb person) every six hours (Lin 1977).

Some people have complained of nausea, vomiting, diarrhea, and light-headedness. So if you choose to use glycerol as a supplement, try smaller doses initially (<0.5 g/kg body weight, or 0.22 g/lb) to see if it's tolerable. Glycerol is currently a component of many protein bars sold on the market, although the doses in these bars are relatively low (10-15 g per bar).

Gynostemma Pentaphyllum

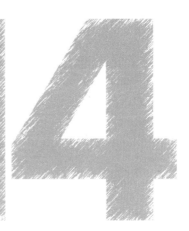

What Is It?

Gynostemma pentaphyllum (GP) is an herb that is commonly grown in China and Japan, and it has been used as food as early as the Ming Dynasty (about 400 years ago). Gypenosides are the active components of GP thought to exert its physiological effects. Gypenosides have a similar structure to ginsenosides, which are the active ingredients in ginseng (Wang et al. 1997; Zhou and Qiu 1990).

How Does It Work?

Gypenosides are very similar in structure to ginsenosides found in ginseng and are believed to have adaptogenic properties; that is, they help the body adapt to various kinds of stress. However, the exact mechanism of action is unknown. This mystery is the problem with ginseng products . . . nobody knows how they work (if indeed they do work at all).

The Evidence: Pro or Con?

In a very limited number of studies, GP has been shown to increase endurance in animals and humans (see table 14.1, but note that only one study has been completed in humans). The data look promising, yet more research is needed to make any conclusions with any confidence.

Table 14.1 Effect of Gynostemma Pentaphyllum Supplementation on Endurance in Mice and Men

Reference	Subjects	Duration	Supplementation	Results
Wang (1997)	15 endurance athletes	30 days	500 mg GP extract PWC_{170} and VO_2	Increase
Zhou (1990)	Mice	18 weeks	3 g GP/kg	39% increase swimming time
Liu (1989)	Mice	3 days	50mg/kg gypenosides	80-111% increase swimming time

Guidelines for Use

There is no concrete support on dosage of GP and at what percent extract of gypenosides. Based on the limited data available, suggested dosage is 500 mg of commercially available GP extract per day for at least 30 days.

Precautions

No known side effects have been reported at 500 mg per day. Future work needs to determine the effects of this plant extract at various doses.

Phosphate

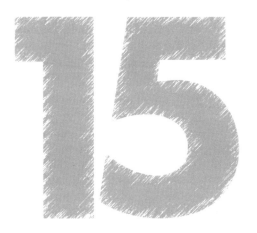

What Is It?

Phosphate (or phosphorus) is a nonmetallic element and, following calcium, is the most abundant mineral in the body. Accordingly, phosphates are important in human metabolism, and they come in different varieties with different functions. For instance, approximately 80 to 90% of the phosphorus in the body combines to form calcium phosphate, which is used for the development of bones and teeth. Phosphate salts, such as sodium phosphate, are involved in acid-base balance. The remainder of the body's phosphates are found in a variety of organic forms, including the phospholipid, which helps form cell membranes and DNA, which is part of the genetic material.

Several other organic phosphates are of prime importance to the athlete. For example, organic phosphates are essential to the normal function of most of the B vitamins involved in the energy processes within the cell. They are also part of the high-energy compounds found in the muscle cell, such as adenosine triphosphate (ATP) and phosphocreatine, which are necessary for muscle contraction. Glucose as well needs to be phosphorylated to proceed through glycolysis, which is a metabolic pathway that produces ATP (energy). Finally, organic phosphates are part of a compound in red blood cells known as 2,3-diphosphoglycerate (2,3-DPG), which facilitates the release of oxygen to the muscle tissues (Williams 1998).

How Does It Work?

Theoretically, phosphate buffers lactic acid, improves the body's ability to deliver oxygen to contracting muscles, and enhances the cardiovascular system's ability to deliver more nutrients to the muscle (Williams 1998). It is believed that supplementing phosphate salts may increase the concentration of 2,3-DPG in red blood cells, which facilitates the release of oxygen to muscles, thus delaying anaerobic glycolysis (lactic acid build-up) and would result in improved endurance performance.

The Evidence: Pro or Con?

The use of phosphate is not a new concept. Phosphate salt supplements, such as sodium and potassium phosphate, were reported to relieve fatigue in German soldiers during World War I (Bucci 1993). In fact, research conducted in Germany during the 1930s suggests that phosphate salts actually improve physical performance. Well-designed, con-

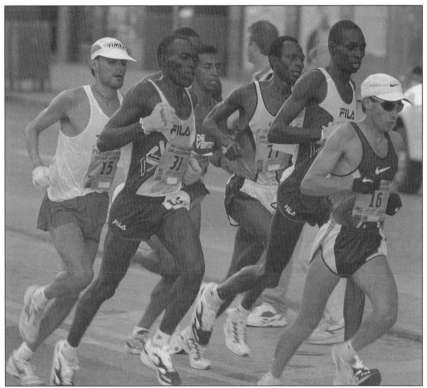

© Human Kinetics

temporary studies are in agreement, as well. Bucci (1993) and Williams (1998) also conclude that phosphate salts may enhance exercise performance.

Dr. Robert Cade and his associates (1984) conducted one of the earliest studies in the United States on phosphate loading at the University of Florida. In a double-blind, placebo-controlled, crossover study, highly trained runners took 1 g sodium phosphate (phosphate salts) four times daily for six days. The phosphate salts increased the concentration of 2,3-DPG in red blood cells by 6.6%, which resulted in an increase in $\dot{V}O_2$max. Remember, the 2,3-DPG facilitates the release of oxygen to muscles, increasing the ability to perform powerful contractions and thus sustain them. Dr. Cade also demonstrated that the amount of lactate produced during a standard exercise workload was lower, and a reduced sensation of physiological stress was also noted during exercise.

In a more recent study, Dr. Richard Kreider and colleagues (1990), using highly trained cross-country runners as subjects, found that 1 g sodium phosphate (phosphate salts) four times daily for six days resulted in 10% increases in $\dot{V}O_2$max and 11.8% in anaerobic threshold. This gain was almost identical to the improvement noted in Dr. Cade's study. Dr. Kreider and colleagues suggested that the improvement in exercise performance was due to increased metabolic efficiency; that is, the body is better at making energy with the aid of sodium phosphate.

Contrary to Dr. Kreider and Dr. Cade, scientists at Brigham Young University found no effect of phosphate supplementation on exercise performance (Duffy and Conlee 1986). Researchers used a double-blind, crossover study with 11 male subjects who underwent the following: acute dosing, 1.24 g sodium and potassium phosphate immediately before exercise; and chronic dosing, 3.73 g/day for six days before exercise testing. Both the short- and long-term phosphate supplementation had no effect on any of the exercise measurements—the two- to three-minute run to exhaustion, isokinetic power, and recovery.

One criticism about this study was that is was designed to study the effects of phosphate salt supplementation on the *anaerobic* energy systems (energy made without oxygen) and not *aerobic* energy systems (energy made with oxygen). Most scientists studying phosphates think that the latter would have been more appropriate to determine any ergogenic effects (Williams 1998). Thus, it seems that sodium phosphates may have an ergogenic effect for endurance athletes while a combination of sodium and potassium phosphates may not. It isn't clear why this is so, but it is a clear illustration that the various types of phosphates affect the body differently.

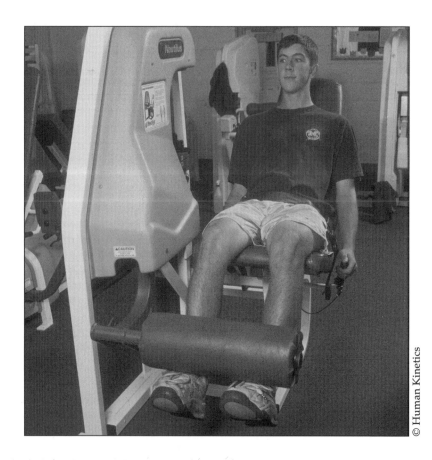

© Human Kinetics

Guidelines for Use

For endurance events such as the 1-mile run or 10 K run, the available data suggest that 1 g sodium phosphate four times a day for six days would be recommended (Cade et al. 1984; Kreider et al. 1990). Less than that would have no effect. Keep in mind that sodium phosphate is different than potassium phosphate. Sodium phosphate seems to have an ergogenic effect; potassium phosphate appears to have none.

Precautions

Daily doses of sodium phosphate (phosphate salts) that do not exceed 4 g appear to be safe, but too much phosphate salt may cause nausea, cramps, and diarrhea. Long-term, high dosing of phosphate salts may impair calcium balance in the body (Williams 1998).

Phosphatidylserine 16

What Is It?

Phosphatidylserine (PS) is a type of lipid (or fat) that is found primarily in cell membranes. Not only is phosphatidylserine important for the normal structure of cell membranes, but some scientists also believe that it is involved in "neuronal excitability, message transduction, and neurotransmitter activity" (Monteleone et al. 1990). In other words, phosphatidylserine may have an effect on neural and endocrine responses. As a supplement, phosphatidylserine became available in the 1990s, and the phosphatidylserine available over the counter is currently derived from soy.

How Does It Work?

Physical stress is associated with an increase in plasma ACTH (adrenocorticotropic hormone), cortisol (the "stress hormone"), growth hormone, prolactin, and lactate with no effect on blood glucose. Treatment with phosphatidylserine can blunt the increase in ACTH and cortisol seen during exercise. Does this mean phosphatidylserine has an "anti-stress" effect and does this translate into an ergogenic effect?

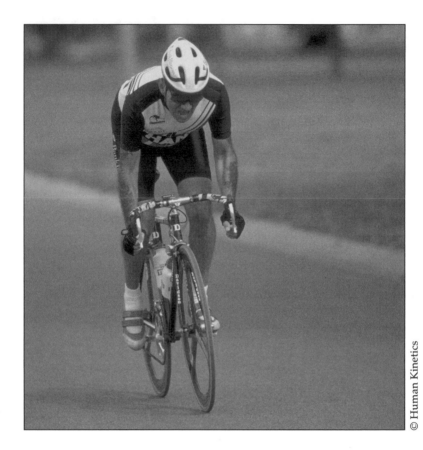

© Human Kinetics

The Evidence: Pro or Con?

To our knowledge, there are only two published studies on the use of PS. In a study published in 1990, Monteleone et al. studied eight healthy men who underwent three experiments with a bicycle ergometer. At 10 to 15 minutes before the start of exercise, subjects received an intravenous infusion of BC-PS (brain-cortex-derived phosphatidylserine) at a dose of 0 (placebo), 50, or 75 mg. Blood samples collected before and after exercise showed that the 75 mg dose had a significant effect on various physiological parameters. When the high dose BC-PS was taken, plasma ACTH and cortisol increased much less. This experiment suggests that phosphatidylserine can partially counteract the release of stress hormones.

In a second experiment, the same group of scientists (Monteleone et al. 1992) examined the effects of 10 days of PS treatment (400 or 800 mg/day, taken orally). During 80 minutes of bicycle exercise, participants who ingested 400 mg/day demonstrated no significant effects; however, PS did blunt the increase of plasma ACTH and cortisol in the subjects who had doses of 800 mg/day. According to these investigators, " . . . chronic oral administration of phosphatidylserine may counteract stress-induced activation of the hypothalamic-pituitary-adrenal axis in man."

Guidelines for Use

Although there are numerous studies showing that PS may prevent the age-related decline in memory and learning (Crook et al. 1991), it isn't clear that this nutrient has a helpful effect in athletics. Thus, recommended doses for athletes have yet to be suggested, but there are suggestions for the nonathletic purposes. According to Dr. Julian Whitaker (1999), "The recommended starting dosage of PS (phosphatidylserine) is 200 to 300 mg daily, tapering down to 100 mg after one month." Keep in mind, though, that this recommendation is not based on PS having any sort of ergogenic effect and is, in our opinion, sheer speculation.

Precautions

There are no known side effects to ingesting PS. Although there is little evidence suggesting that PS might enhance exercise performance, there is plenty of evidence that suggests PS might improve various cognitive disorders. So if you do choose to use it as a "brain booster," we recommend that you consult your physician first.

Polylactate

What Is It?

Polylactate is semisoluble amino acid/lactate salt, and it has been developed as a supplement for increasing endurance performance.

How Does It Work?

Researchers have proposed that polylactate increases pH and bicarbonate levels. If this is truly the case, polylactate would therefore increase the body's ability to buffer lactate in the blood, which in turn could delay the onset of fatigue during exercise and thus improve performance.

The Evidence: Pro or Con?

The future of polylactate as an endurance supplement does not look promising based on the few studies that have been done about its potential as an ergogenic aid. In one study, five trained male cyclists performed on a cycle ergometer three times for 180 minutes at 50% of $\dot{V}O_2$max (Fahey et al. 1991). At 5 minutes before exercise and at 20-minute intervals during exercise, each subject consumed one of the following: a solution containing polylactate (80% polylactate and 20% sodium lactate in 7% solution with water), a glucose polymer (maltodextrin in 7% solution with water), or a control (water sweetened with aspartame).

There were no differences among treatments in perceived exertion, sodium, potassium, chloride, lactate, heart rate, $\dot{V}O_2$max, or body temperature. Polylactate and the glucose polymer, however, produced similar

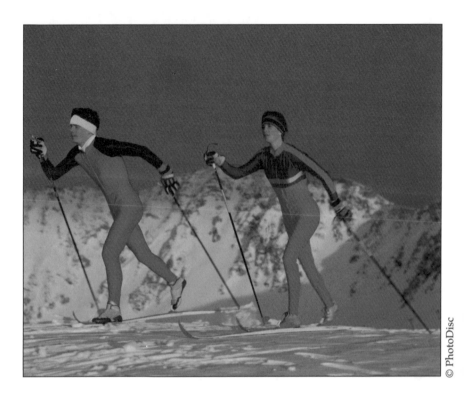

© PhotoDisc

results with the exception that the polylactate increased pH and bicarbonate levels. The authors therefore speculated that polylactate may help maintain blood glucose and enhance blood-buffering capacity during endurance exercise.

In another experiment conducted a few years later, Dr. Swensen and colleagues (1994) conducted a randomized, double-blind study on polylactate using five subjects. The subjects consumed either a glucose polymer solution alone or with polylactate at a rate of 0.3 g carbohydrate per kg body weight (about 0.14 g per lb, or 28 g for a 200-lb person) in a 7% solution every 20 minutes until exhaustion. The glucose polymer–polylactate solution was mixed at a ratio of 6.25 g glucose polymer to 0.75 g polylactate per 100 ml water.

The subjects exercised to exhaustion at 70% $\dot{V}O_2$max before and after supplementation. Oxygen consumption rate, heart rate, and perceived exertion were measured at 20-minute intervals. Serum glucose, insulin, free fatty acids, glycerol, whole blood lactate, and pH were measured at 30-minute intervals. The results showed no significant physiological or performance effects with the addition of polylactate. The researchers concluded that adding polylactate to an energy drink didn't produce any additional performance benefits.

Guidelines for Use

As we mentioned, polylactate has been proposed as a blood buffer. But with only a few studies about its effect on endurance, it is difficult to determine whether it has any performance benefits. Even the few studies that have been conducted on its use have not shown positive results in any aspect. Therefore, until more research shows positive results, we do not recommend polylactate as any sort of endurance supplement.

Precautions

Within the few studies that have been done on the use of polylactate supplementation, even fewer have been done on the issue of safety. In the study by Dr. Swenson and colleagues (1994), subjects ingested polylactate at concentrations greater than 2.5%, and as a consequence, they experienced severe gastrointestinal efflux. The researchers discovered that polylactate ingestion was only tolerable in concentrations of less than 0.75%. We have already illustrated that polylactate is an ineffective ergogenic aid. If one has to experience gastrointestinal upset with its use, it therefore becomes an even more irrelevant supplement.

Protein

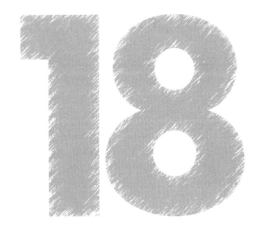

What Is It?

All proteins are composed of amino acids, but there are many different kinds: contractile protein in skeletal muscle; cytoskeletal (or structural) protein in skeletal muscle; enzymes, as components of cells and cell membranes; and hormones, to name a few. The best sources of dietary protein (those with all of the essential amino acids) include milk, egg, whey, casein, beef, chicken, and fish. Soy protein is the only nonanimal source that is of high quality.

How Does It Work?

Proteins are not classically considered a fuel source like fat and carbohydrates; but under certain conditions, protein can be used as a significant source of energy, such as when muscles are glycogen depleted or when the body is suffering from starvation. Endurance athletes often have a misconception that dietary protein is not as important as carbohydrates, but nothing could be further from the truth. Protein helps to repair damaged muscle fibers and promote recovery, and as stated earlier, is used for energy, which usually occurs when athletes are in a carbohydrate-depleted state.

The Evidence: Pro or Con?

For endurance athletes, the recommended daily allowance (RDA) of 0.8 g/kg (0.36g/lb) body weight per day is too low (that's about 72 g for a

Table 18.1 Protein/Energy Needs of Endurance Athletes

	Endurance athlete
Body weight (kg)	60.0
Recommended protein, g/kg body weight	1.4
Total protein, g/day	84.0
Kcal/kg body weight	44.0
Total kcal/day	2,640.0

Data from Williams 1998.

200-lb person). According to Lemon (1998), "Those undergoing endurance training might need 1.2 to 1.6 g/kg (0.54 to 0.73 g/lb) body weight daily (1.5 times the current RDA)" (see table 18.1). In other words, for endurance athletes who weigh 200 lb, they would have to eat between 110 g and 146 g protein.

It may be obvious why strength-power athletes need to consume additional protein (for gaining skeletal muscle mass), but it isn't as apparent why endurance athletes should. Granted, if you eat well—that is, consume fibrous vegetables, starchy carbohydrates, and a lean protein source at each major meal—the need for protein supplementation may be unwarranted. Nonetheless, we do know that prolonged endurance exercise stimulates amino acid oxidation and that protein balance is usually restored after exercise (assuming adequate intake of energy and protein). Therefore, you can lose body mass and protein if you increase exercise demands without a concomitant increase in energy and protein intake.

For many endurance athletes, there is simply no need to carry large amounts of skeletal muscle mass. A cursory look at the elite marathon and ultramarathon competitors reveals a physique that is quite low in body fat and also quite low in skeletal muscle mass. Regarding these athletes, consuming enough calories is more of a critical issue than trying to get adequate protein. With the high-energy intakes required by these athletes, it would seem plausible that they would also meet their protein requirements.

Guidelines for Use

Consuming protein in excess of the RDA is not harmful to healthy, athletic individuals (see following section). Endurance athletes should try to consume roughly 1.5 g protein per kg body weight daily (about 0.7 g protein

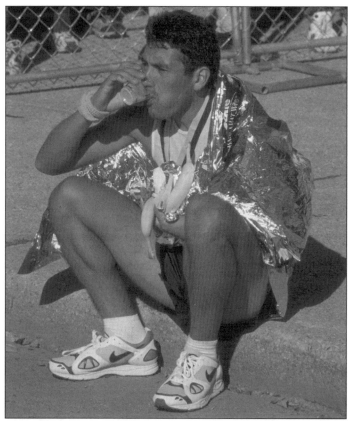

© Human Kinetics

per lb, or 140 g for a 200-lb person). This protein intake can be met with a varied diet. As we mentioned, the best sources of protein include beef, chicken, fish, and pork. However, if you do not eat enough complete protein sources, a variety of meal replacement powders (MRPs) and drinks contain high-quality protein. Most of these MRPs use combinations of whey, casein, or soy protein.

The ideal postworkout meal would be a combination of carbohydrates, protein, and fat (see "Carbohydrate" chapter, page 26). Consuming approximately 1.0-1.5 g carbohydrate per kg (0.5 to 0.7 g CHO/lb) body weight immediately postexercise and 1 hour postexercise is important to meet the needs of glycogen replenishment (assuming, of course, that you eat regular mixed meals [i.e., carbohydrate, protein, and fat] throughout the day). Furthermore, we recommend adding protein (0.5 g per kg [0.23 g/lb] body weight) to those meals to provide the needed amino acids for skeletal muscle repair and recovery. For a 154-lb (70-kg) athlete, this would be 105 g carbohydrate and 35 g protein, met by eating two cups of cooked white rice with a large chicken breast (roasted). Alternatively, meal replacement supplements could also meet these protein needs.

Precautions

There is no evidence that for normal, healthy people, consuming large quantities of dietary protein is harmful. In one study, Poortmans and Dellalieux (2000) studied the effects of a high- and medium-protein intake in bodybuilders and other well-trained athletes and found no harm from eating high quantities of protein. Subjects underwent blood and urine sampling and kept a seven-day food record. Despite higher plasma concentrations of uric acid and calcium, the bodybuilders on the high-protein diet had normal renal clearance of creatinine, urea, and albumin. Interestingly, the nitrogen balance for both groups became positive when daily protein intake exceeded 1.26 g/kg body weight (0.57 g/lb or about 114 g for a 200-lb person). The researchers concluded that daily protein intake under 2.8 g/kg body weight (1.3 g/lb, or 260 g for a 200-lb person) does not appear to "impair renal function in well-trained athletes as indicated by the measures of renal function used in this study."

In an intriguing animal study, Zaragoza et al. (1987) fed rats a diet of 80% protein for more than half of their life span. They found no harmful effects of this high intake of protein. Recently, in an ironic twist, Petzke et al. (2000) sought to "prove" that eating high-protein diets (at least in rats) was harmful. These investigators compared adequate (13.8%), medium (25.7%), and high (51.3%) levels of crude protein intake in rats. What they found was the opposite; it didn't harm the rats. They concluded that "long-term intake of high protein diets did not increase variables of oxidative stress, in contrast with our initial hypothesis."

Another purported health risk of high-protein consumption includes an increased rate of calcium excretion. This is completely overblown. According to a study published in the *Journal of Bone Mineral Research* (Hannan et al. 2000), "Lower protein intake was significantly related to bone loss at the femoral (hip) and spine bone mineral density sites." They state that "higher intake of animal protein does not appear to affect the skeleton adversely." To conclude, there is simply no evidence that shows high-protein intake (twice the RDA) is detrimental to one's health.

Pyruvate

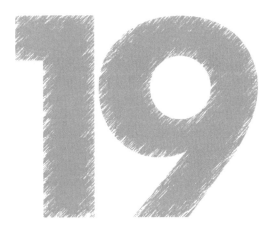

What Is It?

Pyruvate is the end product of glycolysis, which is the body's process of breaking down glucose (sugar) for energy. During the last step in glycolysis, you typically end up with pyruvate, and with the help of oxygen, it is transported into the mitochondria were it is converted into energy (ATP) for muscle contraction. When glycolysis proceeds very quickly (e.g., when you sprint), a lot of that pyruvate is eventually converted to lactate.

How Does It Work?

Some scientists have theorized that when you supplement with pyruvate, the Krebs cycle performs more efficiently, which would lead to an increased rate of ATP production; thus, pyruvate would improve endurance performance by ultimately providing more energy. Studies performed on rats have shown that supplementation with pyruvate lowers the animals' respiratory exchange ratio (Stanko and Adibi 1986), and this mechanism would also lead to an increase in performance. Many studies have been done on pyruvate supplementation and weight loss, but unfortunately, few have been performed on pyruvate's effect on endurance performance. We will examine the current studies in an attempt to glean some possible conclusions.

The Evidence: Pro or Con?

Stanko et al. (1990a) took 10 physically active males and for seven days substituted 25 g pyruvate and 75 g dihydroxyacetone for the same amount of carbohydrate in a standard diet: 55% carbohydrate, 15% protein, 30% fat; 35 kcal/kg body weight (about 16 kcal/lb, or 3,200 kcal for a 200-lb person). An isocaloric glucose polymer solution was used as a placebo. Subjects were tested on an arm ergometer at 60% $\dot{V}O_2$max until exhaustion.

The pyruvate group demonstrated greater endurance than the placebo group (160 minutes vs. 133). These investigators believed that an increase in glucose extraction accounted for the significant increase in arm endurance. For instance, glycogen levels at rest were significantly higher during the pyruvate trial. Additionally, whole arm arteriovenous glucose differ-

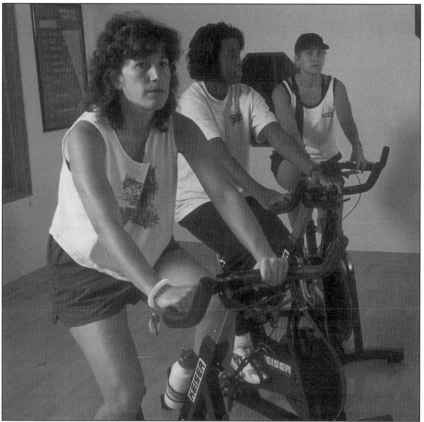

© Human Kinetics

ence was greater at rest and after 60 minutes of exercise, but it did not differ at exhaustion for the supplemented trial versus the placebo.

These same investigators (Stanko et al. 1990b) supplemented eight untrained subjects for seven days with either 100 g polycose (placebo) or dihydroxyacetone (75 g) and pyruvate (25 g) substituted for a portion of carbohydrate in a high-carbohydrate diet: 70% carbohydrate, 18% protein, 12% fat; 35 kcal/kg (about 16 kcal/lb, or 3,200 kcal for a 200-lb person). After the diet, cycle ergometry was performed at 70% $\dot{V}O_2$max until exhaustion. Muscle glycogen at rest and exhaustion did not differ between trials, but time to exhaustion was greater under the pyruvate condition (79 minutes vs. 66). Estimated total glucose oxidation during exercise was significantly greater in the pyruvate group when compared with the placebo, which would again suggest that pyruvate enhances one's ability to utilize glucose for fuel.

A criticism of these studies is that the dose used is tremendously high. It would certainly be unfeasible to consume over 20 grams of pyruvate on a daily basis. In a recent study published in the *Journal of Applied Physiology* (Morrison, Spriet, and Dyck 2000), eight women and one man consumed 7, 15, and 25 g pyruvate to see how much of it appeared in blood. Oddly, they failed to detect any increase in blood pyruvate. They attributed these readings to the possibility that pyruvate is absorbed into circulation but is rapidly cleared (taken up) by muscle or the liver. They stated that "very high concentrations of systemically infused pyruvate are necessary to increase muscle content and that low oral dosages are likely ineffective."

They then tested the effects of seven days of pyruvate supplementation (7 g/day) in seven well-trained cyclists ($\dot{V}O_2$max of 62 ml/kg/minute). When the subjects cycled at 74-80% of $\dot{V}O_2$max, they found no effect on time to exhaustion—91 minutes placebo versus 88 minutes pyruvate (see figure 19.1). Accordingly, the researchers stated that "our results indicate that oral pyruvate supplementation does not increase blood pyruvate content and does not enhance performance during intense exercise in well-trained cyclists."

Using a unique measure of performance, a group from the University of Nebraska-Lincoln examined the effects of pyruvate supplementation on what they referred to as "critical power (CP)" (Ebersole et al. 2000). The CP test "provides an estimate of a power output that can be maintained without fatigue." Researchers used a double-blind, random design with nine male and nine female university crew members assigned to either a placebo or pyruvate treatment. Subjects ingested the supplement (8.1 g/day) for 14 days. Researchers found no effect on "endurance capacity as measured by the CP test."

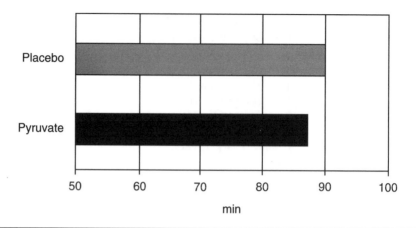

Figure 19.1 When pyruvate supplementation is used with reasonable doses (7-25 g), time to exhaustion is unaffected and pyruvate in the blood is virtually undetected. Data from Morrison, Spriet, and Dyck 2000.

Guidelines for Use

Unless you plan to take over 20 g pyruvate, it will likely have no effect on endurance performance. In the commercially marketed range of 6 g or less, pyruvate is not an ergogenic aid for endurance athletes. Thus, we do not recommend taking this supplement to enhance endurance performance.

Precautions

Supplementation with pyruvate has been shown to have minimal side effects: borborygmous (bowel rumbling), flatus, and diarrhea (Morrison, Spriet, and Dyck 2000; Stanko et al. 1990; Stanko, Tietze, and Arch 1992a, 1992b). Morrison, Spriet, and Dyck (2000) reported that "all subjects complained of borborygmous and flatulence after the 15 g and 25 g trials, indicating pyruvate decarboxylation and the production of gas." Vital functions, blood count, and biochemical profiles are not affected by pyruvate.

Sodium Citrate

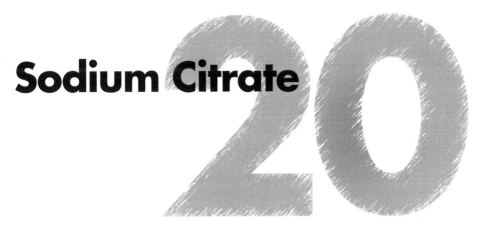

What Is It?

Citrate is a Krebs cycle intermediate and can be found in many common foods such as citrus fruits. The Krebs cycle is basically a way for your body to generate metabolites that are involved in the production of energy (adenosine triphosphate, or ATP). There are numerous "intermediates" in this process and citrate is one of them.

How Does It Work?

Although sodium citrate is not actually a base, it can increase blood pH without the gastrointestinal distress often caused by sodium bicarbonate (Van Someren et al. 1998). Researchers believe that sodium citrate breaks down into bicarbonate in the blood, which ultimately increases the extracellular pH (Tiryaki and Atterbom 1995). If this truly were the case, this process would then provide an artificial way for athletes to their raise extracellular pH and as a consequence maintain the neutral environment necessary for performance.

The questions you may be asking yourself are, why is the ability to increase pH important, and how exactly does it relate to performance? This entire mechanism is made possible through the increased pH difference that is created between the muscle and blood (Cox and Jenkins 1994). During high-intensity exercise, anaerobic glycolysis continually produces H+ ions, which decrease the pH in the muscle cells. Once ingested, the sodium citrate gets into the bloodstream, and the pH in the blood thereby increases. The pH difference then induces an accelerated movement of

H+ ions out of the working muscle tissue and into the extracellular spaces, which consequently raises the intracellular pH (Ibanez et al. 1995). This intracellular increase in pH reduces the negative effects of lactic acid (low pH) and thus allows athletes to perform longer before the onset of fatigue.

The Evidence: Pro or Con?

In exercise lasting between 2 and 15 minutes, sodium citrate supplementation has been shown to have a success rate in improving exercise performance when taken 90 minutes before high-intensity exercise in doses of 0.5 g/kg body weight (about 0.23 g/lb body weight, or 46 g for a 200-lb person) (Linossier et al. 1997; McNaughton and Cedaro 1992). Furthermore, Hausswirth et al. (1995) reported a significant improvement (about 20% greater) in leg endurance when subjects were supplemented with a lower dose of sodium citrate (0.4 g/kg body weight, or 0.18 g/lb) before maximal isometric knee extension. In fact, the most recent study demonstrated that sodium citrate may even improve high-intensity running endurance in elite athletes (Shave et al. 2001). Nine Olympic male and female athletes were given either sodium citrate (0.5 g/kg body weight, or 0.23 g/lb) or placebo dissolved in 1 liter of flavored water 90 minutes before a time trial of 3,000 m (about 3,300 yd). The results illustrated that sodium citrate decreased time by a mean of 10.7 seconds (see figure 20.1).

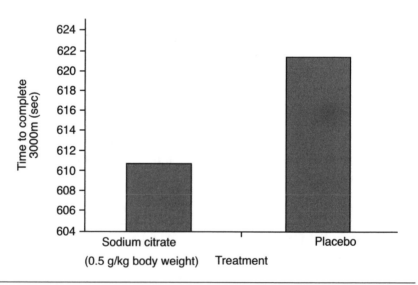

Figure 20.1 Effect of sodium citrate supplementation on a time trial of 3,000 m. Adapted from Shave et al. 2001.

Guidelines for Use

The dose and timing of sodium citrate supplementation should be tested during practice before any major sporting event to ensure tolerability and effectiveness. In our opinion, a single dose of 0.5 g/kg body weight (about 0.23 g/lb body weight, or 46 g for a 200-lb person) diluted in 1 liter of flavored water given 90 minutes before high-intensity endurance exercise (lasting for more than 2 minutes and up to 15 minutes) may result in the greatest benefit on performance. Smaller doses would have no ergogenic effect.

Precautions

One of the advantages sodium citrate may have over other buffers, such as sodium bicarbonate, is that it is well tolerated by most users, as very few subjects have reported gastrointestinal distress during the use of sodium citrate (McNaughton 1990). It should not be overlooked that nausea was one of the main explanations as to why sodium citrate showed no ergogenic potential in the study done by Cox and Jenkins (1994), in which seven of the eight subjects experienced severe nausea. An abundance of water could help ease the gastrointestinal discomfort experienced during sodium citrate ingestion (Cox and Jenkins 1994).

Glossary

ADP (adenosine diphosphate)—An essential chemical involved in the energy production of a cell. ADP is formed when ATP is broken down to supply energy for muscular contraction.

aerobic—Meaning "requiring oxygen." Aerobic metabolism predominates during low-intensity, long-duration exercises.

amino acids—A group of nitrogen-containing, carbon-based organic compounds that serve as the building blocks from which proteins (and muscle) are made.

anabolic—Referring to something that causes a buildup of tissue, or an anabolism. Anabolism generally refers to an increase in lean tissue, particularly muscle.

anaerobic—Anaerobic metabolism involves creating energy (ATP) without oxygen during explosive activities like weightlifting.

anaerobic glycolysis—Refers to the rapid breakdown of glucose or glycogen resulting in the production of energy and an accumulation of lactate.

anti-catabolic—Referring to something that may prevent the breakdown of tissue (muscle).

antioxidants—May help control the damaging effects of free radicals.

anti-proteolysis—This is a specific type of anti-catabolism: namely, the slowing or halting of protein (muscle) breakdown in the body.

ATP (adenosine triphosphate)—High-energy molecule stored in muscle and other cells in the body. When a muscle cell needs energy to contract, ATP is broken down to ADP to provide this energy. ATP can be thought of as the actual fuel that makes muscles move.

benign prostatic hypertrophy—Also known as BPM, refers to the growth of the prostate gland in men; it is commonly seen in men over 50 years. It is a progressive condition that may result in the obstruction of the urethra.

bioavailability—The ease with which something is absorbed from the digestive tract. The higher the bioavailability, the greater the total absorption and rate of absorption.

blind study—A single-blind study is one in which the investigator knows the treatment that each subject receives; however, the subject is unaware of the treatment. A double-blind study is one in which neither the investigator or subject is aware of the treatment.

body mass—Used synonymously with body weight.

body weight—The gravitational force exerted on an object by the force of gravity. Measured in kilograms.

bpm—Beats per minute; the number of times your heart beats in one minute.

buffer—A substance that minimizes changes in hydrogen-ion concentration (pH), such as sodium phosphate that athletes use to help reduce lactic-acid build-up during strenuous exercise.

carbohydrates—Organic compounds containing carbon, hydrogen, and oxygen. A very effective fuel source for the body; each gram contains four calories. Types of carbohydrates include starches, sugars, and fibers. Carbohydrates are classified into three groups: monosaccharides, disaccharides, and polysaccharides. Glucose (blood sugar) is a carbohydrate used by every cell in the body as fuel.

cardiac arrhythmias—Irregular heart beats.

catabolism—Refers to a decrease in lean tissue, particularly muscle.

catecholamines—Refer to the hormones epinephrine and norepinephrine. The catecholamines elevate heart rate, ventilation, etc.

cholesterol—A type of lipid that is a vital component in the production of many steroid hormones in the body; most widely known as a "bad fat," implicated in promoting heart disease and stroke.

coenzyme—An organic compound (contains hydrogen and carbon) that binds to a specific type of enzyme to activate it. A coenzyme is a type of cofactor. B vitamins commonly act as coenzymes.

cofactor—An inorganic substance that binds to a specific type of enzyme to activate it. Vitamins and minerals frequently serve as cofactors.

complete proteins—Proteins that contain all the essential amino acids.

creatine kinase (CK)—CK is an enzyme involved in the transfer of a phosphate between PCr and ADP, thus forming ATP. CK is also leaked from damaged muscle cells and is an indirect measure of muscle fiber injury.

creatine phosphate (CP)—CP donates the energy and the inorganic phosphate molecule that binds with ADP to form ATP. Supplementing with creatine monohydrate helps increase your muscle's CP reserves.

crossover study—A study in which all subjects receive all treatments (i.e., the placebo and the treatment).

deficiency—A suboptimal level of one or more nutrients that are essential for good health. Most often seen with vitamins, a deficiency can be caused by poor nutrition or increased bodily demands, especially from intense training.

dextrose—Another name for glucose.

dipeptides—Protein fragments made up of only two amino acids.

disaccharide—A carbohydrate compound made up of two sugars.

double-blind—A research technique where subjects and researchers do not know who is receiving the experimental supplement or placebo.

efficacy—The maximum ability of a supplement to produce a desired result.

electrolytes—Substances that, in solution, are capable of conducting electricity. These charged particles are present throughout the body and are involved in many activities such as regulating the distribution of water inside and outside cells in the body.

endogenous—Originating from within the body; anything produced inside the body. For example, the hormone testosterone is produced endogenously by the testes in men.

endurance—Muscular endurance is the ability to performance repeated submaximal contractions for a given time period.

enzyme—A protein molecule that acts as a "helper" in thousands of chemical reactions in the body, such as digestion of food, hormone and energy production, and muscle-cell repair.

ergogenic—Possessing the ability to enhance work output, particularly as it relates to athletic performance.

ergolytic—Possessing the ability to decrease work output. Sometimes what is intended to enhance physical performance inadvertently hinders performance.

exogenous—Referring to substances orally consumed that the body endogenously produces.

fat—One of the macronutrients. Fat contains nine calories per gram; it is the most energy-dense macronutrient. Dietary fats may also be referred to as lipids or triglycerides. Fats serve a variety of functions in the body. For example, they act as structural components for all cell membranes, as well as supply necessary chemical substrates for hormone production. There are two types of fat— saturated ("bad") and unsaturated ("good").

fat-free mass (FFM)—All portions of body tissues not containing fat, such as bones, muscles, skin, organs, in addition to body water, hair, blood, and lymph.

free fatty acid levels—Refers to the concentration of fatty acids in plasma (blood).

free form amino acid—Refers to free standing amino acids. In contrast to the amino acids found in proteins.

free radicals—A highly reactive atom or compound having an unpaired electron. Free radicals are produced during metabolism (energy creation) and are believed to cause cellular damage. Free radicals may play a role in aging and disease.

fructose—The main type of sugar found in fruit. Sweeter than table sugar, it is often used as a sugar substitute for diabetics.

glucagon—A hormone that is responsible for helping maintain proper blood sugar levels by breaking down glycogen to glucose.

glucose—The most important carbohydrate in body metabolism. In your body's tissues, glucose may be converted into glycogen, utilized to form fat, or oxidized to carbon dioxide and water.

glucose disposal agent—A nutrient or complex of nutrients that has the ability to increase insulin sensitivity, thus allowing circulating blood glucose to be readily deposited into target tissues.

glycemic index (GI)—A measure of the extent to which a food raises the blood sugar (glucose) level as compared to a standard (usually glucose or white bread).

glycogen—The principal storage form of carbohydrate energy (glucose), which is stored in muscles and in the liver.

glycogenolysis—Refers to the breakdown or degradation of glycogen (the storage form of carbohydrate in liver and muscle).

growth hormone (GH)—An anabolic hormone naturally released by the pituitary gland. GH promotes muscle growth and the breakdown of body fat for energy.

HDL—Stands for "high-density lipoprotein." It's one of the subcategories of cholesterol, typically thought of as the "good" cholesterol.

hematocrit—The percentage of total blood volume that is composed of red blood cells or RBCs; it averages 47% in men and 42% in women.

hormones—Molecules, either protein or steroids, that regulate various biological processes in the body.

hyperthyroidism—A condition caused by excessive secretion of thyroid hormone from the thyroid glands; results in elevation of basal metabolic rate.

hypoglycemia—A condition in which blood glucose is abnormally low.

insulin amplifier—A nutrient or complex of nutrients that has the ability to increase the secretion of insulin.

insulin—An anabolic hormone secreted by the pancreas that aids the body in maintaining proper blood sugar levels and promoting glycogen storage. Insulin secretion speeds the movement of nutrients through the bloodstream and into muscle for growth.

isocaloric—Same number of calories. Thus, if two drinks are isocaloric, it means they have equal calories.

Krebs cycle—Metabolic pathway in the mitochondria in which energy is transferred from carbohydrates, fats, and amino acids to NAD (nicotinamide adenine dinucleotide, a substance involved in the production of energy) for production of ATP.

lactate dehydrogenase (LDH)—An enzyme that catalyzes the oxidation of lactate.

lactic acid—A molecule produced from glucose during anaerobic metabolism. When oxygen becomes available, lactic acid can be completely oxidized or broken down to carbon dioxide and water. Lactic-acid build-up is one cause of muscle fatigue. Supplements that limit lactic-acid build-up may enhance athletic performance.

LDL—Stands for "low-density lipoprotein" and is a subcategory of cholesterol, typically thought of as the "bad" cholesterol. LDL is the type of cholesterol that circulates throughout the bloodstream and may cause heart disease.

lean body mass (LBM)—Another term that describes fat-free mass.

lipid—Another name for dietary fats or triglycerides.

lipogenic—Literally translated as "fat producing"; that is, it means to make body fat.

lipolysis—The chemical breakdown of body fat by enzymes that results in stored body fat being used as fuel by the body.

long-chain fatty acids—Refers to fatty acids that are 12-20 carbons in length.

macronutrient—Refers to carbohydrates, proteins, or fats.

meal-replacement powders (MRPs)—A category of supplements that contain protein, carbohydrates, vitamins, minerals, and other key nutrients. They are used to replace a regular-food meal for purposes of weight loss, weight gain, or increasing dietary nutrient intake.

metabolic rate—The rate of energy utilization by your body. In other words, it's how fast your "whole system" runs. The metabolic rate is controlled by a number of factors such as muscle mass (the greater your muscle mass, the greater your metabolic rate), caloric intake, exercise, and use of stimulant or depressant chemicals.

metabolite—Any product of metabolism, such as an intermediate or waste product. For example, the popular supplement HMB is a metabolite, or breakdown product, of the amino acid leucine.

monoamine oxidase inhibitor (MAOI)—Also known as MAO inhibitors, refers to a group of drugs used to treat depression.

neurotransmitter—Substances released from nerve endings (e.g., acetylcholine) that are involved in a number of biological processes.

nitrogen—An element that distinguishes proteins from other substances and allows them to form various structural units in our bodies, including enzymes and muscle proteins.

nitrogen balance—When a person's daily intake of nitrogen from proteins equals the daily excretion of nitrogen.

nutrients—Components of food that help nourish the body; that is, they provide energy or serve as "building materials." These nutrients include carbohydrates, fats, proteins, vitamins, minerals, water, and so on.

peptide—A compound made up of two or more amino acids. Protein molecules are broken down into peptides in the gut and absorbed in that form.

placebo—A harmless, "inactive" substance that may be given in the place of an effective drug or substance, especially to "control groups" in clinical studies.

placebo-controlled trial—A study in which a placebo (a substance that looks, tastes, and is otherwise not distinguishable from the "real" treatment) is compared to a "real" drug or supplement.

polymer—Refers to a chain of molecules.

polysaccharides—Carbohydrates containing a large number of "sugar groups." Starch, glycogen, dextrin, and cellulose are examples.

power—The amount of work an individual can perform in a given period of time.

precursors—Compounds from which another compound is formed in the body. For example, choline is a precursor to acetylcholine, a neurotrasmitter involved in muscle contraction.

proteins—Highly complex nitrogen-containing compounds found in all animal and vegetable tissues. They are made up of amino acids and are essential for growth and repair in the body. A gram of protein contains four calories. Those from animal sources are high in biological value because they contain essential amino acids. Those from vegetable sources contain some but not all of the essential amino acids. Proteins are the building blocks of muscle, enzymes, and some hormones.

protein-sparing effect—Refers to anti-catabolism.

proteolysis—Breakdown of protein (i.e., catabolism).

pure—Referring to a supplement that contains nothing but the ingredients stated on the label. This term has no legal definition.

randomized study—Refers to studies, in which subjects are randomly assigned to a group (e.g., coin toss) to be studied. For instance, if you have 100 subjects, you would randomly assign them to group A or B via a coin toss.

saturated fats—"Bad" fats. They are called "saturated" because they contain no open spots on their "carbon skeletons." Saturated fats include myristic acid, palmitic acid, stearic acid, and arachadonic acid, which have been shown to raise cholesterol levels in the body. Sources of these fats include animal foods and hydrogenated vegetable oils, such as margarine. These fats serve no biological function in the body, other than to supply calories.

sucrose—Most commonly known as table sugar. Industrially, sucrose is derived from sugar cane or sugar beets. When you eat it, the body breaks sucrose into fructose and glucose; consequently, it has some of the properties of fructose and some of the properties of glucose. Eating it elicits a rapid insulin response, but not as high as one caused by glucose.

thermogenic—Meaning speed up the metabolism, raise core body temperature, and accelerate calorie expenditure.

triglyceride—The scientific name for a common dietary fat. The backbone of this molecule is a glycerol molecule that is connected to three fatty acid molecules. Triglycerides are also called fats or lipids.

unsaturated fats—"Good" fats. They are called unsaturated because they have one or more open "carbon spots." Unsaturated fats can be divided into two categories: polyunsaturated fats and monounsaturated fats. Unsaturated fats have been shown to help reduce cholesterol and triglyceride levels in the blood. This category of fats includes the essential fatty acids linoleic acid and alpha-linolenic acid.

vitamins—Organic compounds that are vital to life, indispensable to bodily function, and needed in minute amounts. They are noncaloric essential nutrients. Many of them function as coenzymes, supporting a multitude of biological functions.

$\dot{V}O_2$max—The maximum volume of oxygen an individual can consume per minute of work. It is often used to evaluate an athlete's aerobic power (i.e., cardiac output, oxygen-extracting ability).

References

Allen, J.D., J. McLung, A.G. Nelson, and M. Welsch. 1998. Ginseng supplementation does not enhance healthy young adult's peak aerobic exercise performance. *Journal of American College of Nutrition* 17:462-466.

Antonio, J., and C. Street. 1999. Glutamine: A potentially useful supplement for athletes. *Canadian Journal of Applied Physiology* 24:1-14.

Aphale, A.A., A.D. Chhibba, N.R. Kumbhakarna, M. Maeenuddin, and S.H. Dahat. 1998. Subacute toxicity study of the combination of ginseng (Panax ginseng) and ashwagandaha (Withania somnifera) in rats: a safety assessment. *Indian Journal of Physiology and Pharmacology* 42:299-302.

Bahrke, M.S., and W.P. Morgan. 2000. Evaluation of the ergogenic properties of ginseng. *Sports Medicine* 29:113-133.

Balsom, P.D., S.D. Harridge, K. Soderlund, B. Sjodin, and B. Ekblom. 1993. Creatine supplementation per se does not enhance endurance exercise performance. *Acta Physiological Scandinavia* 149 (4):521-523.

Bangsbo, J., P.D. Gollnick, T.E. Graham, et al. 1990. Anaerobic energy production and O_2 deficit-debt relationship during exhaustive exercise in humans. *Journal of Physiology (London)* 422:539-559.

Bell, D.G., and I. Jacobs. 1999. Combined caffeine and ephedrine ingestion improves run times of Canadian Forces Warrior Test. *Aviation, Space, and Environmental Medicine* 70 (4):325-328.

Bell, D.G., I. Jacobs, T.M. McLellan, and J. Zamecnik. 2000. Reducing the dose of combined caffeine and ephedrine preserves the ergogenic effect. *Aviation, Space, and Environmental Medicine* 71 (4):415-419.

Bell, D.G., I. Jacobs, T.M. McLellan, M. Miyazaki, and C.M. Sabiston. 1999. Thermal regulation in the heat during exercise after caffeine and ephedrine ingestion. *Aviation, Space, and Environmental Medicine* 70 (6):583-587.

Bessman, S.P. 1986. The physiological significance of the creatine phosphate shuttle. *Advance Experimental and Medical Biology* 194:1-11.

Bessman, S.P. 1987. The creatine phosphate energy shuttle: The molecular asymmetry of a "pool." *Annals of Biochemistry* 161 (2):519-523.

113

Bishop, P.A., J.F. Smith, and B. Young. 1987. Effects of N, N-Dimethylglycine on physiological response and performance in trained runners. *Journal of Sports Medicine* 27:53-56.

Black, D.G., and A.A. Sucec. 1981. Effects of calcium pangamate on aerobic and endurance parameters, a double-blind study. *Medicine and Science in Sports and Exercise* 13:93.

Blomstrand, E., P. Hassmen, B. Ekblom, and E.A. Newsholme. 1991. Administration of branched-chain amino acids during sustained exercise-effects on performance and plasma concentration of some amino acids. *European Journal of Applied Physiology* 63:83-88.

Blomstrand, E., P. Hassmen, S. Ek, et al. 1997. Influence of ingesting a solution of branched-chain amino acids on perceived exertion during exercise. *Acta Physiologica Scandinavica* 159:41-49.

Blomstrand, E., S. Andersson, P. Hassmen, et al. 1995. Effect of branched-chain amino acid and carbohydrate supplementation on the exercise-induced change in plasma and muscle concentration of amino acids in human subjects. *Acta Physiologica Scandinavica* 153:87-96.

Blumenthal M., W.R. Busse, A. Goldberg, et al., eds. 1998. *The complete commission E monographs: Therapeutic guide to herbal medicines.* Boston: Integrative Medicine Communications.

Bonetti, A., et al. 2000. Effect of ubidecarenone oral treatment on aerobic power in middle-aged trained subjects. *Journal of Sports Medicine and Physical Fitness* 40:51-57.

Boza, J.J., et al. 2001. Effect of glutamine supplementation of the diet on tissue protein synthesis rate of glucocorticoid-treated rats. *Nutrition* 17:35-40.

Braun, B., P.M. Clarkson, P.S. Freedson, and R.L. Kohl. 1991. Effects of coenzyme Q10 supplementation on exercise performance, $\dot{V}O_2$max, and lipid peroxidation in trained cyclists. *International Journal of Sport Nutrition* 1 (4):353-365.

Brown, R.C., and C.M. Cox. 2000. High fat versus high-carbohydrate diets: Effect on exercise capacity and performance of endurance trained cyclists. *New Zealand Journal of Sports Medicine* 28:55-59.

Brown, R.C., and C.M. Cox. 2001. Challenging the dogma of dietary carbohydrate requirements for endurance athletes. *American Journal of Medicine and Sports* 3:75-86.

Bucci, L. 1993. *Nutrients as ergogenic aids for sports and exercise.* Boca Raton, FL: CRC Press.

Buckley, J., et al. 1998. Effect of oral bovine colostrurm supplement (Intact) on running performance. *Proceedings of the Australian Conference of Science and Medicine in Sport* (October):79.

Buckspan, R., B. Hoxworth, E. Cersosimo, J. Devlin, E. Horton, and N. Abumrad. 1986. A-Ketoisocarpoate is superior to leucine in sparing glucose utilization in man. *American Journal of Physiology* 251:E648-E653.

Burke, L.M., et al. 1998. Carbohydrate intake during prolonged cycling minimizes the effect of glycemic index of pre-exercise meal. *Journal of Applied Physiology* 85:2220-2226.

Burke, L.M., et al. 2000. Carbohydrate loading failed to improve 100-km cycling performance in a placebo-controlled trial. *Journal of Applied Physiology* 88:1284-1290.

Burke, L. www.sportsci.org. Carbohydrate Intake Targets for Athletes: Grams or Percent? Australian Institute of Sport, Camberra, Australia.

Cade, R., M. Conte, et al. 1984. Effects of Phosphate loading on 2,3-diphosphoglycerate and maximum oxygen uptake. *Medicine and Science in Sports and Exercise* 16:263-268.

Castell, L.M., and E.A. Newsholme. 1998. Glutamine and the effects of exhaustive exercise upon the immune response. *Canadian Journal of Physiology and Pharmacology* 76:524-532.

Castell, L.M., J.R. Poortmans, and E.A. Newsholme. 1996. Does glutamine have a role in reducing infections in athletes? *European Journal of Applied Physiology* 73:488-490.

Cerosimo, E., B.M. Miller, W.W. Lacy, and N. Abrumrad. 1983. A-Ketoisocaproate, not leucine, is responsible for nitrogen sparing during progressive fasting in normal male volunteers. *Surgical Forum* 34:96-98.

Chesley, A., R.A. Howlett, G.J.F. Heigenhauser, E. Hultman, and L.L. Spriet. 1998. Regulation of muscle glycogenolytic flux during intense aerobic exercise after caffeine ingestion. *American Journal of Physiology* 275:596-602.

Chua, B., D.L. Siehl, and H.E. Morgan. 1979. Effect of leucine and metabolites of branched chain amino acids on protein turnover in heart. *Journal of Biological Chemistry* 254:8358-8362.

Clarkson, P.M., and H.S. Thompson. 1997. Drugs and sports research findings and limitations. *Sports Medicine* 24 (6):367-381.

Colombani, P., C. Wenk, I. Kunz, et al. 1996. Effects of L-carnitine supplementation on physical performance and energy metabolism of endurance-trained athletes: A double-blind placebo crossover field study. *European Journal of Applied Physiology* 73:434-439.

Coombes, J.S., and L.R. McNaughton. 2000. Effects of branched-chain amino acid supplementation on serum creatine kinase and lactate dehydrogenase after prolonged exercise. *Journal of Sports Medicine and Physical Fitness* 40(3):240-246.

Costill, D.L., G.P. Dalsky, and W.J. Fink. 1978. Effects of caffeine ingestion on metabolism and exercise performance. *Medicine and Science in Sports and Exercise* 10:155-158.

Cox, G., and D.G. Jenkins. 1994. The physiological and ventilatory responses to repeated 60s sprints following sodium citrate ingestion. *Journal of Sports Sciences* 12:469-475.

Crook, T.H., J. Tinklenberg, J. Yesavage, et al. 1991. Effects of phosphatidylserine in age-associated memory impairment. *Neurology* 41:644-649.

Daniels, J.W., P.A. Mole, J.D. Shaffrath, and C.L. Stebbins. 1998. Effects of caffeine on blood pressure, heart rate, and forearm blood flow during dynamic leg exercise. *Journal of Applied Physiology* 85:154-159.

Demant, T.W., and E. Rhodes. 1999. Effects of creatine supplementation on exercise performance. *Sports Medicine* 28 (1):49-60.

Dodd, S.L., E. Brooks, S.K. Powers, and R. Tulley. 1991. The effects of caffeine on graded exercise performance in caffeine naïve versus habituated subjects. *European Journal of Applied Physiology* 62:424-429.

Duffy, D.J., and R.K. Conlee. 1986. Effects of phosphate loading on leg power and high intensity treadmill exercise. *Medicine and Science in Sports and Exercise* 18:674-677.

Dunagan, N., J.E. Greenleaf, and C.J. Cisar. 1998. Thermoregulatory effects of caffeine ingestion during submaximal exercise in men. *Aviation, Space, and Environmental Medicine* 69 (12):178-181.

Earnest, C.P., A.L. Almada, and T.L. Mitchell. 1997. Effects of creatine monohydrate ingestion upon intermediate length anaerobic treadmill running to exhaustion. *Journal of Strength and Conditioning Research* 4:234-238.

Ebersole, K.T., J.R. Stout, J.M. Eckerson, T.J. Housh, T.K. Evetovich, and D.B. Smith. 2000. The effect of pyruvate supplementation on critical power. *Journal of Strength and Conditioning Research* 14 (2):132-134.

Edwards, M., E. Rhodes, D. McKenzie, and A. Belcastro. 2000. The effect of creatine supplementation on anaeorbic performance in moderately active men. *Journal of Strength and Conditioning Research* 14 (1): 75-79.

Engels, H.J., and J.C. Wirth. 1997. No ergogenic effects of ginseng (Panax ginseng C.A. Meyer) during graded maximal aerobic exercise. *Journal of the American Diet Association* 97:1110-1115.

Erickson, M.A., et al. 1987. Effects of caffeine, fructose, and glucose ingestion on muscle glycogen utilization during exercise. *Medicine and Science in Sports and Exercise* 19 (6):579-583.

Fahey, T.D., J.D. Larsen, G.A. Brooks, W. Colvin, S. Henderson, and D. Lary. 1991. The effects of ingesting polylactate or glucose polymer drinks during prolonged exercise. *International Journal of Sports Nutrition* 1:149-156.

Falk, B., R. Burstein, J. Rosenblum, Y. Shapiro, E. Zylber-Katz, and N. Bashan. 1990. Effects of caffeine ingestion on body fluid balance and thermoregulation during exercise. *Canadian Journal of Pharmacology* 68:889-892.

Febbraio, M., et al. 2000a. Effects of carbohydrate ingestion before and during exercise on glucose kinetics and performance. *Journal of Applied Physiology* 89:2220-2226.

Febbraio, M.A., et al. 2000b. Pre-exercise carbohydrate ingestion, glucose kinetics, and muscle glycogen use: Effect of the glycemic index. *Journal of Applied Physiology* 89:1845-1851.

Febbraio, M., T. Flanagan, R. Snow, S. Zhao, and M. Carey. 1995. Effect of creatine supplementation on intramuscular TCr, metabolism and performance during intermittent, supramaximal exercise in humans. *Acta Physiological Scandinavian* 155:387-395.

Fisher, S.M., R.G. McMurray, M. Berry, M.H. Mar, and W.A. Forsythe. 1986. Influence of caffeine on exercise performance in habitual caffeine users. *International Journal of Sports Medicine* 7:276-280.

Frayn, K.N., K. Khan, S.W. Coppack, et al. 1991. Amino acid metabolism in human subcutaneous adipose tissue in vivo. *Clinical Science* 80:471-474.

Gallagher, P.M., J.A. Carrithers, M.P. Godard, K.E. Schulze, and S. W. Trappe. 2000a. β-hydroxy-β-methylbutyrate ingestion, part I: Effects on strength and fat free mass. *Medicine and Science in Sports and Exercise* 32:2109-2115.

Gallagher, P.M., J.A. Carrithers, M.P. Godard, K.E. Schulze, and S. W. Trappe. 2000b. β-hydroxy-β-methylbutyrate ingestion, part II: Effects on hematology, hepatic and renal function. *Medicine and Science in Sports and Exercise* 32:2116-2119.

Gascon, G., B. Patterson, K. Yearwood, and H. Slotnick. 1989. N, N-dimethyglycine and epilepsy. *Epilepsia* 30:90-93.

Gilliam, J., C. Hohzorn, D. Martin, and M. Trimble. 2000. Effect of oral creatine supplementation on isokinetic torque production. *Medicine and Science in Sports and Exercise* 32 (5):993-996.

Gillis, C.N. 1997. Panax ginseng pharmacology: A nitric oxide link? *Biochemistry Pharmacology* 54:1-8.

Girandola, R.N., R.A. Wiswell, and A. Bulbulian. 1980. Effects of pangamic acid (B-15) ingestion on metabolic response to exercise. *Biochemistry Medicine* 24:218-222.

Gorostiaga, E.M., C.A. Maurer, and J.P. Eclache. 1989. Decrease in respiratory quotient during exercise following L-carnitine supplementation. *International Journal of Sports Medicine* 10:169-174.

Graham, T.E., and L.L. Spriet. 1995. Metabolic, catecholamine, and exercise performance responses to various doses of caffeine. *Journal of Applied Physiology* 78 (3):867-874.

Graham, T.E., E. Hibbert, and P. Sathasivam. 1998. The metabolic and exercise endurance effects of coffee and caffeine ingestion. *Journal of Applied Physiology* 85:883-889.

Gray, M.E., and L.W. Titlow. 1982. B15: Myth or miracle. *Physicians Sports Medicine* 10:107-112.

Greig, C., K.M. Finch, D.A. Jones, et al. 1987. The effect of oral supplementation with L-carnitine on maximum and submaximum exercise capacity. *European Journal of Applied Physiology* 56:457-460.

Hannan, M.T., K.L. Tucker, B. Dawson-Hughes, et al. 2000. Effect of dietary protein on bone loss in elderly men and women: The Framingham Osteoporosis Study. *Journal of Bone Mineral Research* 15:2504-2512.

Hargreaves, M., and R. Snow. 2001. Amino acids and endurance exercise. *International Journal of Sport Nutrition and Exercise Metabolism* 11:133-145.

Harris R.C., M. Viru, P.L. Greenhaff, and E. Hultman. 1993. The effect of oral creatine supplementation on running performance during maximal short term exercise in man. *Journal of Physiology (London)* 467:74P.

Hausswirth, C., A.X. Bigard, R. Lepers, M. Berthelot, and C.Y. Guezennec. 1995. Sodium citrate ingestion and muscle performance in acute hypobaric hypoxia. *European Journal of Applied Physiology* 71:362-368.

Herbert, B. 1979. Pangamic acid (Vitamin B15). *American Journal of Clinical Nutrition* 32:1534-1540.

Horvath, P.J., et al. 2000. The effects of varying dietary fat on performance and metabolism in trained male and female runners. *Journal of the American College of Nutrition.* 19(1):52-60.

Hu, F.B., J.E. Manson, and W.C. Willett. 2001. Types of dietary fat and risk of coronary heart disease: A critical review. *Journal of the American College of Nutrition* 20:5-19.

Hunt, S.M., and J.L. Groff. 1990. *Advanced nutrition and human metabolism.* St. Paul: West.

Ibanez, J., T. Pullinen, E. Gorostiaga, A. Postigo, and A. Mero. 1995. Blood lactate and ammonia in short-term anaerobic work following induced alkalosis. *The Journal of Sports Medicine and Physical Fitness* 35:187-193.

Iyer, R.N., A.A. Khan, A. Gupta, et al. 2000. L-carnitine moderately improves the exercise tolerance in chronic stable angina. *The Journal of the Association of Physicians of India* 48:1050-1052.

Jacobs, I., S. Bleue, and J. Goodman. 1997. Creatine ingestion increases anaerobic capacity and maximum accumulated oxygen deficit. *Canadian Journal of Applied Physiology* 22:231-243.

Kamikawa, T., A. Kobayashi, T. Yamashita, H. Hayashi, and N. Yamazaki. 1985. Effects of coenzyme Q10 on exercise tolerance in chronic stable angina pectoris. *American Journal of Cardiology* 56 (4):247-251.

Kemp, G.L. 1959. A clinical study and evaluation of pangamic acid. *Journal of American Osteopathic Association* 58:714.

Kern, P.A., M.E. Svoboda, R.H. Eckel, and J.J. Van Wyk. 1989. Insulin-like growth factor action and production in adipocytes and endothelial cells from human adipose tissue. *Diabetes* 38:710-717.

King, R., C.B. Cooke, and J. O'Hara. 2001. The use of galactose in sports drinks before exercise. *The FASEB Journal* 15:A990 (abstract no. 756.4).

Kirwan, J.P., D. O'Gorman, and W.J. Evans. 1998. A moderate glycemic meal before endurance exercise can enhance performance. *Journal of Applied Physiology* 84:53-59.

Kishikawa, Y., et al. 1996. Purification and characterization of cell growth factor in bovine colostrum. *Journal of Veterinarian Medicine Science* 58:47-53.

Knitter, A.E., L. Panton, J.A. Rathmacher, A. Petersen, and R. Sharp. 2000. Effects of β-hydroxy-β-methylbutyrate on muscle damage after a prolonged run. *Journal of Applied Physiology* 89:1340-1344.

Kreider, R.B., D. Hill, G. Horton, M. Downes, S. Smith, and B. Anders. 1995. Effects of carbohydrate supplementation during intense training on dietary patterns, psychological status, and performance. *International Journal of Sport Nutrition* 5:125-135.

Kreider, R.B., G.W. Miller, M.H. Williams, C.T. Somma, and T.A. Nasser. 1990. Effects of phosphate loading on oxygen uptake, ventilatory anaerobic threshold, and run performance. *Medicine and Science in Sports and Exercise* 22:250-256.

Kuhne, S., et al. 2000. Growth performance, metabolic and endocrine traits, and absorptive capacity in neonatal calves fed either colostrum or milk replacer at two levels. *Journal of Animal Science* 78:609-620.

Kuipers, H., et al. 2001. Colostrum has no effect on growth factors and on a doping test. *Medicine and Science in Sports and Exercise* 33 (5):S338.

Labow, B.I., and W.W. Souba. 2000. Glutamine. *World Journal of Surgery* 24:1503-1513.

Lacey, J.M., and D.W. Wilmore. 1990. Is glutamine a conditionally essential amino acid? *Nutrition Reviews* 48:297-309.

Lambert, E.V., et al. 1994. Enhanced endurance in trained cyclists during moderate intensity exercise following 2 weeks adaptation to a high fat diet. *European Journal of Applied Physiology* 69:287-293.

Langenfeld, M.E., J.G. Seifert, S.R. Rudge, and R.J. Bucher. 1994. Effect of carbohydrate ingestion on performance of non-fasted cyclists during a simulated 80-mile time trial. *Journal of Sports Medicine and Physical Fitness* 34:263-270.

Laurent, D., K.E. Schneider, W.K. Prusaczyk, C. Franklin, S.M. Vogel, M. Krssak, K.F. Petersen, H.W. Goforthe, and G.I. Shulman. 2000. Effects of caffeine on muscle glycogen utilization and the neuroendocrine axis during exercise. *The Journal of Clinical Endocrinology Society* 85 (6):2170-2174.

Lemon, P.W. 1998. Effects of exercise on dietary protein requirements. *International Journal of Sport Nutrition* 8:426-447.

Lemon, P.W., et al. 1997. Moderate physical activity can increase dietary protein needs. *Canadian Journal of Applied Physiology* 22 (5):494-503.

Levenhagen, D.K., J.D. Gresham, M.G. Carlson, et al. 2001. Postexercise nutrient intake timing in humans is critical to recovery of leg glucose and protein homeostasis. *American Journal of Physiology, Endocrinology and Metabolism* 280:E982-E993.

Lin, E.C. 1977. Glycerol utilization and its regulation in mammals. *Annual Review of Biochemistry* 46:765-795.

Linossier, M.T., D. Dormis, P. Bregere, A. Geyssant, and C. Denis. 1997. Effect of sodium citrate on performance and metabolism of human skeletal muscle during supramaximal cycling exercise. *European Journal of Applied Physiology* 76:48-54.

Liu, X. S., J. Gan, and R.B. Huang. 1989. Pharmacological study of Gypenosides of Gynostemma Pentaphyllum (Thunb) Makino from Guang Xi province. *Chinese Traditional Patent Medicine* 11 (8):27-29.

Loster, H., K. Miehe, M. Punzel, O. Stiller, H. Pankau, and J. Schauer. 1999. Prolonged oral L-carnitine substitution increases bicycle ergometer performance in patients with severe, ischemically induced cardiac insufficiency. *Cardiovascular Drugs and Therapy* 13 (6):537-546.

Ludwig, D.S., et al. 1999. High glycemic foods, overeating, and obesity. *Pediatrics* 103:E26.

Lyons, T.P., M.L. Riedesel, L.E. Meuli, and T.W. Chick. 1990. Effects of glycerol-induced hyperhydration prior to exercise in the heat on sweating and core temperature. *Medicine and Science in Sports and Exercise* 22:477-483.

MacLean, D.A., T.E. Graham, and B. Saltin. 1994. Branched-chain amino acids augment ammonia metabolism while attenuating protein breakdown during exercise. *American Journal of Physiology* 267:E1010-E1022.

Marconi, C., G. Sassi, A. Carpinelli, and P. Ceretelli. 1985. Effects of L-carnitine loading on the aerobic and anaerobic performance of endurance athletes. *European Journal of Applied Physiology* 54:131-135.

McArdle, W.D., F.I. Katch, and V.L. Katch. 1999. *Sports & Exercise Nutrition.* Baltimore: Lippincott Williams & Wilkins.

McNaughton, L., and R. Cedaro. 1992. Sodium citrate ingestion and its effects on maximal anaerobic exercise of different durations. *European Journal of Applied Physiology* 64:36-41.

McNaughton, L.R. 1990. Sodium citrate and anaerobic performance: Implications of dosage. *European Journal of Applied Physiology* 61:392-397.

Mero, A., et al. 1997. Effects of bovine colostrum supplementation on IGF-1, IGG and saliva IGA during training. *Journal of Applied Physiology* 83:1144-1151.

Millard-Stafford, M., L.B. Rosskopf, T.K. Snow, and B.T. Hinson. 1994. Pre-exercise carbohydrate-electrolyte ingestion improves one-hour running performance in the heat. *Medicine and Science in Sports and Exercise* 26:S196.

Mitch, W.F., M. Walser, and D.G. Spair. 1981. Nitrogen sparing induced by leucine compared with that induced by its keto-analogue, alpha-ketoisocaproic in fasting, obese man. *Journal of Clinical Investigation* 67:553-562.

Mittleman, K.D., et al. 1998. Branched-chain amino acids prolong exercise during heat stress in men and women. *Medicine and Science in Sports and Exercise* 30(1):83-91.

Monteleone, P., L. Beinat, C. Tanzillo, M. Maj, and D. Kemali. 1990. Effects of phosphatidylserine on the neuroendocrine response to physical stress in humans. *Neuroendocrinology* 52:243-248.

Monteleone, P., M. Maj, L. Beinat, M. Natale, and D. Kemali. 1992. Blunting by chronic phosphatidylserine administration of the stress-induced activation of the hypothalamo-pituitary-adrenal axis in healthy men. *European Journal of Clinical Pharmacology* 41:385-388.

Montner, P., D.M. Stark, M.L. Riedesel, et al. 1996. Pre-exercise glycerol hydration improves cycling endurance time. *International Journal of Sports Medicine* 17:27-33.

Morrison, M.A., L.L. Spriet, and D.J. Dyck. 2000. Pyruvate ingestion for 7 days does not improve aerobic performance in well-trained individuals. *Journal of Applied Physiology* 89:549-556.

Mortimore, G.E., A.R. Poso, M. Kadowaki, and J.J. Wert. 1987. Multiphasic control of hepatic protein degradation by regulatory amino acids, general features and hormonal modulation. *Journal of Biological Chemistry* 262:16322-16327.

Muoio, D.M., J.J. Leddy, P.J. Horvath, A.B. Awad, and D.R. Pendergast. 1994. Effect of dietary fat on metabolic adjustments to maximal $\dot{V}O_2$ and endurance runners. *Medicine and Science for Sports and Exercise* 26:81-88.

Murray, R., D.E. Eddy, G.L. Paul, J.G. Seifert, and G.A. Halaby. 1991. Physiological responses to glycerol ingestion during exercise. *Journal of Applied Physiology* 71:144-149.

Nelson, A., R. Day, E. Glickman-Weiss, M. Hegstad, and B. Sampson. 2000. Creatine supplementation alters the response to a graded cycle ergometer test. *European Journal of Applied Physiology* 83 (1):89-94.

Nicholas, C.W., C. Williams, G. Phillips, and A. Nowitz. 1996. Influence of ingesting a carbohydrate-electrolyte solution on endurance capacity during intermittent, high intensity shuttle running. *Journal of Sports Science* 13:283-290.

Niles, E.S., et al. 2001. Carbohydrate-protein drink improves time to exhaustion after recovery from endurance exercise. *Journal of Exercise Physiology* 4 (1):45-52.

Nissen, S., R. Sharp, M. Ray, J. Rathmacker, D. Rice, J. Fuller, A. Connelly, and N. Abumrad. 1996. Effect of leucine metabolite β-hydroxy-β-methybutyrate on muscle metabolism during resistance-exercise training. *Journal of Applied Physiology* 81 (5):2095-2104.

Nissen, S., R.L. Sharp, L. Panton, M. Vukovich, S. Trappe, and J.C. Fuller. 2000. β-Hydroxy-β-Methylbutyrate (HMB) supplementation in humans is safe and may decrease cardiovascular risk factors. *Journal of Nutrition* 130:1937-1945.

Noia, G., et al. 1996. Coenzyme Q10 in pregnancy. *Fetal Diagnosis and Therapy* 11 (4):264-270.

Okano, G., Y. Sato, Y. Takumi, and M. Sugawara. 1996. Effect of 4h pre-exercise high carbohydrate and high fat meal ingestion on endurance performance and metabolism. *International Journal of Sports Medicine* 17 (7):530-534.

Oyono-Enguelle, S., H. Freund, C. Ott, et al. 1988. Prolonged submaximal exercise and L-carnitine in humans. *European Journal of Applied Physiology* 58:53-61.

Pakkanen R., and J. Aalto. 1997. Growth factors and antimicrobial factors of bovine colostrum. *International Dairy Journal* 7:285-297.

Pasman, W.J., et al. 1995. The effect of different dosages of caffeine on endurance performance time. *International Journal of Sports Medicine* 16 (4):225-230.

Pawlak, D.B., et al. 2001. High glycemic index starch promotes hypersecretion of insulin and higher body fat in rats without affecting insulin sensitivity. *Journal of Nutrition* 131:99-104.

Pearson, D., D. Hamby, W. Russel, and T. Harris. 1999. Long-term effects of creatine monohydrate on strength and power. *Journal of Strength and Conditioning Research* 13(3):187-192.

Pendergast, D.R., J.J. Leddy, and J.T. Venkatraman. 2000. A perspective on fat intake in athletes. *Journal of the American College of Nutrition* 19 (3):345-350.

Petzke, K.J., A. Elsner, J. Proll, F. Thielecke, and C.C. Metges. 2000. Long-term high protein intake does not increase oxidative stress in rats. *Journal of Nutrition* 130:2889-2896.

Pieralisi, G.P. Ripari, and L. Vecchiet. 1991. Effects of a standardized ginseng extract combined with dimethylaminoethanol bitartrate, vitamins, minerals, and trace elements on physical performance during exercise. *Clinical Therapy* 13:373-382.

Pipes, T.V. 1980. The effects of pangamic acid on performance in trained athletes. *Medicine and Science in Sports and Exercise* 12:98.

Poortmans, J.R., and O. Dellalieux. 2000. Do regular high protein diets have potential health risks on kidney function in athletes? *International Journal of Sport Nutrition and Exercise Metabolism* 10:28-38.

Porter, D.A., et al. 1995. The effect of oral coenzyme Q10 on the exercise tolerance of middle-aged, untrained men. *International Journal of Sports Medicine* 16:421-427.

Powell, T., F.F. Hsu, J. Turk, and K. Hruska. 1998. Ma-huang strikes again: Ephedrine nephrolithiasis. *American Journal of Kidney Disease* 32:153-159.

Prevost, M.C., A.G. Nelson, and G.S. Morris. 1997. Creatine supplementation enhances intermittent work performance. *Research Quarterly for Exercise and Sport* 68:233-240.

Rasmussen, B.B., K.D. Tipton, S.L. Miller, S.E. Wolfe, and R.R. Wolfe. 2000. An oral essential amino acid-carbohydrate supplement enhances muscle protein anabolism after resistance exercise. *Journal of Applied Physiology* 88:386-392.

Reap, E.A., and J.W. Lawson. 1990. Stimulation of the immune response by dimethylglycine, a nontoxic metabolite. *Journal of Laboratory Clinical Medicine* 115:481-486.

Rotman, S., et al. 2000. Muscle glycogen recovery after exercise measured by ^{13}C-magnetic resonace spectroscopy in humans: Effect of nutritional solutions. *Magnetic Resonance Materials in Physics, Biology, and Medicine* 11:114-121.

Rowbottom, D.G., D. Keast, and A.R. Morton. 1996. The emerging role of glutamine as an indicator of exercise stress and overtraining. *Sports Medicine* 21:80-97.

Scaglione, F., G. Cattaneo, M. Alessandria, and R. Cogo. 1996. Efficacy and safety of the standardized ginseng extract G115 for potentiating vaccination against the influenza syndrome and protection against the common cold. *Drugs in Experimental and Clinical Research* 22:65-72.

Shave, R., G. Whyte, A. Siemann, and L. Doggart. 2001. The effects of sodium citrate ingestion on 3,000 meter time-trial performance. *Journal of Strength and Conditioning Research* 15 (2):230-234.

Shimomura, Y., M. Suzuki, S. Sugiyama, Y. Hanaki, and T. Ozawa. 1991. Protective effect of coenzyme Q10 on exercise-induced muscular injury. *Biochemical and Biophysical Research Communications* 176 (1):349-355.

Sinclair, C.J.D., and J.D. Geinger. 2000. Caffeine use in sports a pharmacological review. *The Journal of Sports Medicine and Physical Fitness* 40 (1):71-77.

Smith, J.C., D.P. Stephens, E.L. Hall, A.W. Jackson, and C.P. Earnest. 1998. Effect of oral creatine ingestion on parameters of the work rate-time relationship and time to exhaustion in high-intensity cycling. *European Journal of Applied Physiology* 77 (4):360-365.

Snider, I.P., T.L. Bazzarre, S.D. Murdoch, and A. Goldfarb. 1992. Effects of coenzyme athletic performance system as an ergogenic aid on endurance performance to exhaustion. *International Journal of Sport Nutrition* 2 (3):272-286.

Spriet, L.L., D.A. MaClean, D.J. Dyck, E. Hultmant, et al. 1992. Caffeine ingestions and muscle metabolism during prolonged exercise in humans. *American Journal of Physiology* 262 :E891-E898.

Stackpoole, P.W. 1977. Pangamic acid (Vitamin B15). *World Review for Nutrition and Diet* 27:145-163.

Stanko, R.T., and S.A. Adibi. 1986. Inhibition of lipid accumulation and enhancement of energy expenditure by the addition of pyruvate and dihydroxyacetone to a rat diet. *Metabolism* 35:182-186.

Stanko, R.T., et al. 1990a. Enhancement of arm exercise endurance capacity with dihydroxyacetone and pyruvate. *Journal of Applied Physiology* 68(1):119-124.

Stanko, R.T., R.J. Robertson, R.W. Galbreath, J.J. Reilly, K.D. Greenawalt, and F.L. Gross. 1990b. Enhanced leg exercise endurance with a high carbohydrate diet and dihydroxyacetone and pyruvate. *Journal of Applied Physiology* 69:1651-1656.

Stanko, R.T., D.L. Tietze, and J.E. Arch. 1992a. Body composition, energy utilization, and nitrogen metabolism with a severely restricted diet supplemented with dihydroxyacetone and pyruvate. *American Journal of Clinical Nutrition* 55:771-776.

Stanko, R.T., D.L. Tietze, and J.E. Arch. 1992b. Body composition, energy utilization, and nitrogen metabolism with a 4.25-MJ/d low-energy diet supplemented with pyruvate. *American Journal of Clinical Nutrition* 56:630-635.

Stannard, S.R., et al. 2000. The effect of glycemic index on plasma glucose and lactate levels during incremental exercise. *International Journal of Sport Nutrition and Exercise Metabolism* 10:51-61.

Stout, J., J. Eckerson, K. Ebersole, G. Moore, S. Perry, T. Housh, A. Bull, J. Cramer, and A. Batheja. 2000. Effect of creatine loading on neuromuscular fatigue threshold. *Journal of Applied Physiology* 88:109-112.

Struder, H.K., W. Hollmann, P. Platen, et al. 1998. Influence of paroxetine, branched-chain amino acids and tyrosine on neuroendocrine system responses and fatigue in humans. *Hormone and Metabolic Research* 30:188-194.

Sung, B.H., W.R. Lovallo, T. Whitsett, and M.F. Wilson. 1995. Caffeine elevates blood pressure response to exercise in mild hypertensive men. *American Journal of Hypertension* 8:1184-1888.

Swensen, T., G. Crater, D.R. Bassett, and E.T. Howley. 1994. Adding polylactate to a glucose polymer solution does not improve endurance. *International Journal of Sports Medicine* 15:430-434.

Tarnopolsky, M.A., et al. 1997. Postexercise protein-carbohydrate and carbohydrate supplements increase muscle glycogen in men and women. *Journal of Applied Physiology* 83:1877-1883.

Tarnopolsky, M.A., S.A. Atkinson, J.D. MacDougall, D.G. Sale, and J.R. Sutton. 1989. Physiological responses to caffeine during endurance running in habitual caffeine users. *Medicine and Science in Sports and Exercise* 21:418-424.

Taubes, B. 2001. The soft science of dietary fat. *Science* 291:2536-2545.

The Columbia Encyclopedia, sixth edition. 2001. www.bartleby.com/65/gl/gycerol.html.

Tiryaki, G.R., and H.A. Atterbom. 1995. The effects of sodium bicarbonate and sodium citrate on 600 m running time of trained females. *The Journal of Sports Medicine and Physical Fitness* 35:194-198.

Van Hall, G., J.S. Raaymakers, W.H. Saris, and A.J. Wagenmakers. 1995. Ingestion of branched-chain amino acids and tryptophan during sustained exercise in man: Failure to affect performance. *Journal of Physiology* 486:789-794.

Van Hall, G., S.M. Shirreffs, and J.A.L. Calbet. 2000. Muscle glycogen resynthesis during recovery from cycle exercise: No effect of additional protein ingestion. *Journal of Applied Physiology* 88:1631-1636.

Van Soeren, M.H., and T.E. Graham. 1998. Effect of caffeine on metabolism, exercise endurance, and catecholamine responses after withdrawal. *The American Physiological Society* 85 (4):1493-1500.

Van Someren, K., K. Fulcher, J. McCarthy, J. Moore, G. Horgan, and R. Langford. 1998. An investigation into the effects of sodium citrate ingestion on high-intensity exercise performance. *International Journal of Sport Nutrition* 8:357-363.

Vecchiet, L., F. Di Lisa, G. Pieralisi, et al. 1990. Influence of L-carnitine administration on maximal physical exercise. *European Journal of Applied Physiology* 61:486-490.

Volek, J.S., and W.J. Kraemer. 1996. Creatine supplementation: Its effect on human muscular performance and body composition. *Journal of Strength and Conditioning Research* 10:200-210.

Vukovich, M.D., and G.D. Adams. 1997. Effect of β-hydroxy β-methylbutyrate (HMB) on VO_2 peak and maximal lactate in endurance trained cyclist. *Medicine and Science in Sport and Exercise* 29 (5):S252.

Vukovich, M.D., D.L. Costill, and W.J. Fink. 1994. Carnitine supplementation: Effect on muscle carnitine and glycogen content during exercise. *Medicine and Science in Sports and Exercise* 26:1122-1129.

Wagner, D. 1999. Hyperhydrating with glycerol: Implications for athletic performance. *Journal of the American Dietetic Association* 99:207-212.

Wallimann, T., M. Wyss, D. Brdiczka, K. Nicolay, and H.M. Eppenberger. 1992. Intracellular compartmentation, structure and function of creatine kinase isoenzymes in tissues with high and fluctuating energy demands: The 'phosphocreatine circuit' for cellular energy homeostasis. *Biochemistry Journal* 281 (Pt.1):21-40.

Wang, L.C., and T.F. Lee. 1998. Effect of ginseng saponins on exercise performance in non-trained rats. *Planta Medica* 64:130-133.

Wang, Z.F., K.M. Hu, J.S. Shu, and Y. Wang. 1997. Effects of Rhodiola rosea extract on the fatigue and the endurance in athletes. *Journal of ChengDu University of Traditional Chinese Medicine* 20 (2):35-38.

Watanabe, S., R. Ajisaka, T. Masuoka, et al. 1995. Effects of L- and DL-carnitine on patients with impaired exercise tolerance. *Japanese Heart Journal* 36:319-331.

Wemple, R.D., D.R. Lamb, and K.H. McKeever. 1997. Caffeine vs. caffeine-free sports drinks: Effects on urine production at rest and during prolonged exercise. *International Journal of Sports Medicine* 18:40-46.

Weston, S.B., S. Zhou, R.P. Weatherby, and S.J. Robson. 1997. Does exogenous coenzyme Q10 affect aerobic capacity in endurance athletes? *International Journal of Sport Nutrition* 7 (3):197-206.

Whitaker, J. 1999. *The memory solution.* Garden City, NY: Avery Publishing Group.

White, L.M., S.F. Gardner, B.J. Gurley, et al. 1997. Pharmacokinetics and cardiovascular effects of ma-huang (Ephedra sinica) in normotensive adults. *Journal of Clinical Pharmacology* 37:116–121.

Whitley, H.A., et al. 1998. Metabolic and performance responses during endurance exercise after high-fat and high-carbohydrate meals. *Journal of Applied Physiology* 85(2):418-424.

Willett, W.C. 1998. Is dietary fat a major determinant of body fat? *American Journal of Clinical Nutrition* 67 (suppl):556S-562S.

Williams, M.H. 1998. *The ergogenics edge.* Champaign, IL: Human Kinetics.

Williams, M.R. 2001. *Nutrition for health, fitness, and sport.* New York: McGraw Hill.

Williams, M.R., R.B. Kreider, and D. Branch. 1999. *Creatine: The power supplement.* Champaign, IL: Human Kinetics.

Wyss, V., G.P. Ganzit, and A. Rienzi. 1990. Effects of L-carnitine administration on $\dot{V}O_2$max and the aerobic-anaerobic threshold in normoxia and hypoxia. *European Journal of Applied Physiology* 60:1-6.

Yaspelkis III, B.B., J.G. Patterson, P.A. Anderla, Z. Ding, and J.L. Ivy. 1993. Carbohydrate supplementation spares muscle glycogen during variable-intensity exercise. *Journal of Applied Physiology* 75:1477-1485.

Ylikoski, T., J. Piirainen, O. Hanninen, and J. Penttinen. 1997. The effect of coenzyme Q10 on the exercise performance of cross-country skiers. *Molecular Aspects of Medicine* 18 (supplement):S283-S290.

Zaragoza, R., J. Renau-Piqueras, M. Portioles, et al. 1987. Rats fed a prolonged high protein diet show an increase in nitrogen metabolism and liver megamitochondria. *Archives of Biochemistry and Biophysics* 258 (2):426-435.

Zhou, S.R., and Z.R. Qiu. 1990. A preliminary study on the effects of gynostemma pentaphyllum on endurance, spontaneous motor activity and superoxide dismutase in mice. *Asia Pacific Journal of Pharmacology* 5:321-322.

Ziegler, T.R., et al. 1990. Safety and metabolic effects of L-glutamine administration in humans. *Journal of Parenteral and Enteral Nutrition* 14:137S-146S.

Ziemba A.W., J. Chmura, H. Kaciuba-Uscilko, K. Nazar, P. Wisnik, and W. Gawronski. 1999. Ginseng treatment improves psychomotor performance at rest and during graded exercise in young athletes. *International Journal of Sport Nutrition* 9:371-377.

About the Authors

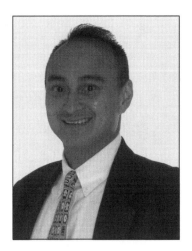

Jose Antonio earned his PhD in muscle physiology from the University of Texas Southwestern Medical Center in Dallas. He has scientific publications in the areas of muscle growth, androgen metabolism, and sports nutrition. Furthermore, he has numerous articles in Muscle & Fitness and other fitness-oriented magazines. His current position is senior manager in sports science for Nutricia. He currently resides in Florida with his wife and twin daughters.

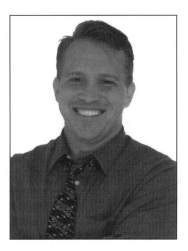

Jeffrey R. Stout earned his PhD in exercise physiology from the University of Nebraska-Lincoln. He has scientific publications in the areas of sports nutrition, muscle fatigue, growth and development, and body composition. Dr. Stout was recently awarded the Outstanding Young Investigator Award and the Editorial Excellence Award by the National Strength and Conditioning Association. He currently resides in Florida with his wife, son and daughter.

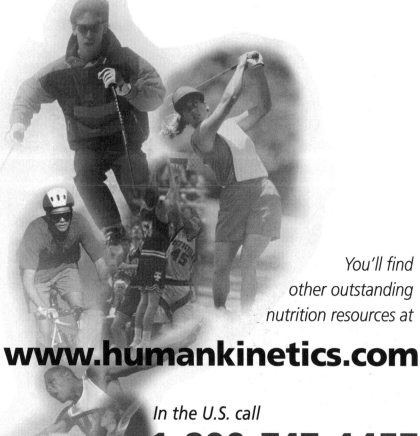